HEALTH PROMOTION AND EXERCISE FOR OLDER ADULTS

An Instructor's Guide

HEALTH PROMOTION AND EXERCISE FOR OLDER ADULTS

An Instructor's Guide

Carole B. Lewis, PT, PhD

Physical Therapy Services of Washington, Inc.
Washington, DC

Linda C. Campanelli, PhD

Professor, Department of Health and Fitness
The American University
Washington, DC

Aspen Series in Physical Therapy
Carole B. Lewis, Series Editor

AN ASPEN PUBLICATION®
Aspen Publishers, Inc.
Gaithersburg, Maryland
1990

Library of Congress Cataloging-in-Publication Data

Lewis, Carole Bernstein. Health promotion and exercise
for older adults : an instructor's
guide / Carole B. Lewis, Linda C. Campanelli.
p. cm.

Includes bibliographical references.
ISBN: 0-8342-0169-0
1. Aged—Health and hygiene. 2. Physical fitness for the aged. 3. Health
promotion. I. Campanelli, Linda C. II. Title. [DNLM: 1. Exercise. 2. Health
Promotion. 3. Physical Fitness. QT 255 L673h]
RA564.8.L47 1990
613'.0438—dc20
DNLM/DLC
for Library of Congress
90-739
CIP

The authors have made every effort to ensure the accuracy of the information
herein, particularly with regard to technique and procedure. However, appropriate information sources should be consulted, especially for new or unfamiliar procedures. It is the responsibility of every practitioner to evaluate the appropriate-
ness of a particular opinion in the context of actual clinical situations and with due
consideration to new developments. Authors, editors, and the publisher cannot be
held responsible for any typographical or other errors found in this book.

Editorial Services: Ruth Bloom

Library of Congress Catalog Card Number: 90-739
ISBN: 0-8342-0169-0

Printed in the United States of America

2 3 4 5

We would like to dedicate this book
to our loving husbands,
Mark Wagner and *Cord Jones*,
who have been supportive and understanding through
the entire process of writing, editing, and publishing.
They have always encouraged us to be active and to
exercise. They have made exercise an important part of
their lives as well.

Table of Contents

Preface

This book is designed to meet what the authors see as a need for a practical, how-to health promotion and exercise manual for allied health professionals who instruct older adults. Both authors have taught exercise classes in the community and have developed stylized classes to simplify the process of facilitating and leading exercise sessions. The exercises in this book have been developed for the nonprofessional, but the seasoned rehabilitation professional who is beginning to work with individual classes can also benefit.

Each chapter addresses a particular area in a step-by-step approach. For example, the first part of each class module includes a lecture/discussion, followed by detailed exercises that are appropriate for older adults. At the end of each module are camera-ready handouts that the instructor can copy to distribute to class participants.

The beginning chapters of this manual cover practical background information, such as how to contract for services with outside agencies, as well as how to set up and lead classes. The manual ends with chapters on special problems and program evaluation.

In summary, this is a practical guide for clinicians who are interested in leading health promotion and exercise classes. We are hopeful that it also will help the clinician to develop health promotion classes as an added tool for rehabilitation efforts in daily practice.

Acknowledgments

Carole Lewis would like to acknowledge Therese McNerney and Kathy Ripley for their assistance in organizing and proofreading portions of the manuscript. Linda Campanelli would like to acknowledge C. Darrell Jones for his assistance in editing, organizing, and preparing portions of the manuscript. Both authors thank Loretta Stock and Nancy Weisgerber of Aspen Publishers, Inc., for their encouragement, and Bob Savannah for his artistic skills used in creating the artwork for this book.

Introduction

The notion that health promotion is an effective approach to retarding aging and maintaining health has finally been accepted. Putting it in perspective, the postulates of compressed morbidity, enhanced plasticity, and the roles of personal decision and personal effort legitimize health promotion efforts. To postpone illness through health promotion has tremendous implications for both the older adult and society as a whole. Functional independence is prolonged while direct caregiving by children to parents or institutionalization of family members is postponed.

Postponing the onset of illness or maintaining current health status is important, as a senior boom is being forecast. With the Baby Boomers (i.e., those born between 1946 and 1964) about to enter young old age, it has been predicted that, in the year 2020, every fourth U.S. citizen could be over 65 years of age. Moreover, the composition of those surviving into older age has changed. When the average American male reaches his 65th birthday, he can expect to live another 11 years. When the average American woman reaches her 65th birthday, she can expect to live another 20 years. Because more people are living

longer, companionship into later life also becomes an issue. The 1980 U.S. census produced the following startling facts: the ratio of men to women at age 50 is 1:1; at age 65 to 74, 77:100; at age 75 to 84, 50:100; and at age 85 and older, 44:100.[1,p3] The implications for older women in particular are astounding.

Issues in health promotion relative to an aging population encompass the individual, the surrounding environment, and the community. Because health promotion is a process that involves the physical, psychological, social, and spiritual aspects of a person's life, the challenge remains to ensure its place among all aspects of medical care, whether in an institution (hospital or nursing home) or at home.

It has often been said that it is discouraging to work with older adults because they may have multiple illnesses, are noncompliant with prescribed medications, or lack an intact support system. It is the belief of the authors that there are barriers to health promotion efforts involving issues of self-efficacy and compliance in all age groups. The nature of health promotion work with older adults, however, requires an inherent belief that such efforts are not in vain and that, with adequate social support and follow-up, functioning can be improved or maintained.

The most challenging barrier to an enhanced quality of life is a lack of motivation to engage in a lifetime of health-related activities. Unfortunately, motivation is not easily understood. That which motivates one individual may turn away another. We are hopeful that our well-organized and focused classes will facilitate the health professional's role as motivator as well as enthuse the participants.

We have written this manual in a format that we believe will be easy to use. Our goals were simple: make it camera-ready for your easy use and make it good. Although we have limited our topics, we have written what we have experienced first-hand and have determined to be most relevant to any health promotion program. Because we were compelled to be brief and to the point, there is plenty of room for your own elaborations on any given topic.

There is no doubt that health promotion activities are the key to the maintenance of function and rehabilitation. This program is both cost-effective to the consumer and the health care system. We've done the hardest part for you. It's your turn to "just do it!"

Note: When working with elderly clients, you may want to increase the size when reproducing the handouts.

NOTE

1. Ken Dychtwald. *Wellness and Health Promotion for the Elderly* (Rockville, Md.: Aspen Publishers, Inc., 1985).

BIBLIOGRAPHY

Fries, J., and L. Crapo. *Vitality and Aging.* San Francisco, W.H. Freeman and Company, 1981.

Part I

Getting Started

1

Why Classes?

The federal government and the public at large continue to scrutinize the cost of rehabilitation. Some people feel that too much is being spent on individual rehabilitation programs. One answer to this is to provide classes for groups of individuals who have been through rehabilitative programs, but still need follow-up treatment, or who have been unable to obtain rehabilitation services. Classes are also viable alternatives for older persons who have been receiving individual rehabilitation services, but have reached a point where their advances are so slow that they do not warrant the cost of individualized physical therapy or occupational therapy intervention. Furthermore, classes can help older persons retain the benefits of rehabilitation for a longer period of time.

When thinking of classes, consider the population. For example, elderly patients who have undergone an amputation, who have arthritis, or who have had a stroke, may be the perfect group to get together for an exercise class. If a group of older patients is simply in need of education or exercise, classes may be an answer. Senior citizens are open to general classes on a variety of rehabilitative problems. An osteoporosis class, for example, may spark interest in older retirement community residents. In

addition, arthritis and balance tend to be of concern to many people as they grow older. Therefore, the attendance in these types of classes is likely to be very good.

An initial concern about classes is payment. One way that some therapists secure funding is to have the facility pay for the classes. A second option is to have the individuals in the class pay a small fee to the therapist. On the other hand, the therapist may decide to conduct classes for good will.

The benefits of conducting classes are numerous. Classes can be a good public relations tool for the health professional who is seeking recognition in the area of geriatric rehabilitation. Classes can improve the therapist's image, helping the nursing staff, nursing home residents, medical staff, and social work staff to perceive the therapist as a helpful and educational person. Another good reason for teaching classes is that, while conducting the class, the leader may be able to screen participants for potential rehabilitation problems. For example, the leader may notice a lack of coordination in an older woman who is attending a balance class. Such a coordination problem may indicate a neurological deficit or muscle strength deficit for which the leader can suggest a specific supervised physical therapy or occupational therapy program. An older man who comes to a posture class may mention during class that he has neck pain. He may accept this pain as "old age." In reality, he may have a treatable condition that would improve with a physical therapy intervention. So conducting exercise classes is a way of providing information on the one hand and evaluating the health status of the community on the other. Finally, classes allow rehabilitation professionals, who generally have an opportunity to provide information only on a one-to-one basis, to reach a broader audience in an extremely cost-effective way.

2

How To Get Started

The most difficult part of any venture is getting started. Fears and apprehensions can keep a potential star from shining. To arrange an exercise class for older persons, take the following steps:

1. Find an appropriate facility.
2. Write a letter.
3. Make a telephone call.
4. Visit and establish a relationship.
5. Write a letter to participants.
6. Put up and/or send out flyers.
7. Check out final preparations.

FACILITIES

A good place to start looking for a facility is where older persons work, live, gather for recreation, meet, or visit. The following may be good places to display or advertise for an exercise class:

- Meeting places of local chapters of the National Retired Teachers Association and the American Association of Retired Persons
- Senior centers or senior citizens centers

- Universities (e.g., adult education or adult health and development programs)
- Retirement centers
- Long-term care facilities
  1. nursing homes
  2. skilled nursing facilities
  3. extended care facilities
- Outpatient rehabilitation departments
  1. hospitals
  2. rehabilitation centers
  3. private offices
- Doctors' offices
  1. internists
  2. rheumatologists
  3. orthopedic surgeons
  4. neurologists
  5. geriatricians
  6. family practitioners
- Health clubs (e.g., any special programs already being offered for the "over 50")

Once you think you have found the place for a class, call and find out who is the administrator, program director, office manager, or owner. Check to be sure its hours, goals, population, and location fit with your agenda. You can get much of this information from a telephone call.

PERSONAL INTRODUCTION

After you have found out who is in charge of the facility, write that person a letter. In the letter, describe yourself and the class. Include your resumé and a list of topics for the classes (Appendix 2-A). Also, tell the person that you plan to call and set up a meeting.

Ms. Ann Jones
Mill Vill Retirement Home
South Pond, WY 12345

Dear Ms. Jones:

My name is Carole Smith, and I am interested in talking to you about setting up some very special exercise classes. My background is in physical therapy, and I have worked for more than 10 years with older people. I would like to share some of my expertise with the members of Mill Vill Retirement Home before they need the individualized services of a physical therapist.

My classes are special because they are on different subjects, such as arthritis, back pain, and neck stiffness, to name just a few.

I have enclosed my resumé as well as a list of topics for the exercise group. Please review the information at your leisure. In the meantime, if you have any questions, I can be reached at 555-1212.

I plan to call you to set up a meeting in a week. Thank you for your time.

Sincerely,

Carole Smith, P.T.

The next week, when you make the telephone call, you may say something like this.

Hello, Ms. Jones. My name is Carole Smith. I wrote to you about a week ago about the possibility of my conducting an exercise class. I was wondering if you would like to get together and discuss this. What is a good time for you? Good, I look forward to seeing you then.

Prior to the visit, decide (1) what fee you are willing to accept and what fee you will ask; (2) how long your class will be (30 to 50 minutes?); (3) how often (e.g., daily, weekly, monthly) the class will meet; (4) what you are willing to provide (e.g., handouts, music, exercise paraphernalia); and (5) what you require (e.g., publicity, guest room, stereo, immediate payment). Prepare a contract (Appendix 2-B), a sample letter to potential class members (Appendix 2-C), and a sample flyer (Appendix 2-D). Armed with these materials, go in and negotiate. The following is a sample visit:

Hi, Ms. Jones. I'm Carole Smith. [Make small talk here; discuss the weather, how nice the facility is.] Did you have a chance to look over the material I sent you? [If not, have an extra copy to give her, and discuss the topics.] Do you think this program would be a welcome addition at Mill Vill? Are you interested? I would like to start doing the class on a weekly basis and see how well it is received. My fee is $100 per class. Is that agreeable to you? Good. I have a contract that I brought to protect both of us. If you will sign it, I can begin in three weeks. In the meantime, I have a letter to your residents to introduce me and get their ideas. If you could pass these out, I will be back in a week to get the responses. Then one week before class, I will come around with flyers announcing the class.

A note on fees—if this is your first class, you may have to ask or accept a lower fee. You may even have to do one or two free sessions. Calculate your fees based on the following: (1) experience in leading classes, (2) the money you could be earning by treating patients, (3) the free public relations (PR) from the class, and (4) the need for exposure and experience. Such a formula might look like this.

Experience (never led a class) =	+ Money for treating patients	− Free PR	+ Need for exposure		FEE
$0	+ $50	− $25	− $25	=	$0 (no charge)
Experience (led many classes) =	+ Money for treating patients	− Free PR	+ Need for exposure		FEE
$100	+ $50	− $25	− $25	=	$100
Experience (led many classes) =	+ Money for treating patients (new in area and not very busy)	− Free PR	+ Need for exposure		FEE
$100	$0	− $40	− $35	=	$ 25

You must estimate the value of the various items. Try the formula for your marketplace, and, if the price is too high or too low, change it.

FINAL PREPARATIONS

Before your first class, be sure to have your handouts run off and your music ready. Go to the facility an hour early. Help set up the room. Check to be sure your tape plays properly.

Then leave a half hour for time to go around to those at the facility and ask if they are coming to the class. Let the administrator know that you are there. Finally, five to ten minutes before class, wait by the door and greet the participants with a handout and a smile as they come into the room.

LIABILITY CONSIDERATIONS

Since we are such a litigious society, it is important for you to consider your personal liability in teaching an exercise class. First, be sure that your insurance policy covers you while you are conducting classes; almost all consulting policies do. If your policy does not cover you, get a new policy. Second, have each participant sign a consent form before your first session (Appendix 2-E). To do this, have a sign-up sheet for class participants. Then either send or ask the staff to distribute these forms. The forms can be collected as each participant enters the room for the first class. A medical release form also helps limit your liability (Appendix 2-F). (Regardless of any forms that the participants sign, the exercise leader *is liable* for any act of negligence.) This form can also be handed out ahead of time. For this form, give the class participants a month either to visit their doctor or to send the doctor the form.

PRE-CLASS EVALUATION

It is not essential to collect information on your class participants. Nevertheless, if later you decide to research and describe your group, having this information can be very resourceful. Appendixes 2-G and 2-H are two examples of initial background forms.

Appendix 2-A

Topic List for Classes

- Fancy Footwork
- Lavish Legs
- Knowledgeable Knees
- Happy Hips
- Better Backs
- Nice Necks
- Supple Shoulders
- Agile Arms
- Wonderful Wrists
- Hardy Hands and Flexible Fingers
- Improving Balance
- Realizing Relaxation
- Abatable Arthritis
- Preventing Parkinson's Problems
- Opposing Osteoporosis
- Perfect Posture
- Getting Stronger
- Better Breathing
- Stopping Stroke
- Ways To Walk
- Facts on Flexibility
- Correcting Coordination
- Understanding Aerobics
- All about Alzheimer's Disease
- Achieving Perfect Body Weight
- Exercising Facial Muscles
- Hidden Exercises

Appendix 2-B

Sample Contract

I, _____contract with

_____ to provide a

_____ exercise/discussion class on various topics.
(frequency)

I agree to bring handouts and cassette tapes. _____ agrees to provide

chairs, stereo, and batons as well as $100.00 (one hundred dollars) per class to be paid within two weeks of the class.

This contract can be terminated with 30 days' notice by either party.

_____	_____
Date	Signature
_____	_____
Date	Signature

Note: An attorney can suggest additions and variations of this sample agreement and should be consulted regarding the full implications of any contractual commitments.

Appendix 2-C

Sample Letter to Potential Class Members

Dear Mill Vill Residents:

Allow me to introduce myself. My name is Carole Smith and I am a physical therapist with 10 years' experience. My specialty is the bone and muscle problems of older people.

On Monday, June 18, from 11:00 to 12:00, I will be leading an exercise class and a brief discussion of osteoporosis. I will be returning to conduct other discussions as well and would like you to help me determine which ones would be of interest to you. Please check those of interest and add any others. Thank you in advance for your help.

See you in exercise class soon!

Sincerely,

Carole Smith, P.T.

Please fill out and return to the front desk.

TOPICS

___ Arthritis	___ Increasing Flexibility
___ Posture	___ Getting Stronger
___ Neck Pain	___ Aerobics—Pros and Cons
___ Relieving Back Pain	___ Stress Management
___ Fixing Shoulder Problems	___ Walking Programs
___ All about Knees	___ Exercises for You
___ Feet Work	___ Helping Hands
___ Improving Balance	___ Better Breathing
___ Correct Coordination	___ Hidden Exercises
___ Walking Better	___ _____

Appendix 2-D

Sample Flyer

OSTEOPOROSIS CLASS

11:00 - 12:00

Monday, June 18th
in the
Dining Room

MEET

Carole Smith, Physical Therapist

LISTEN, LEARN, & EXERCISE

for Osteoporosis
and

HAVE FUN DOING IT!

Appendix 2-E

Participant Consent Form

I understand that the purpose of this (project or program) is to enhance my health-fitness status.

I verify that my participation is fully voluntary, and no coercion of any sort has been used to obtain my participation.

I understand that I may withdraw from the (project or program) without prejudice or malice at any time during the involved period or session.

I have been informed of the procedures and methods that will be used in the (project or program) and understand what will be necessary for me as a participant.

I understand that my participation will remain anonymous unless expressed name permission is given by me.

Signed: _____

Date: _____

Appendix 2-F

Medical Release Form

_____ has my permission to participate in a physical exercise

program to be given at _____. I understand that this

course consists of gentle stretching and strengthening programs of a mild exercise

performance level. I have listed below any problems that the health professional

leading this class should be aware of and that may affect this patient's performance

in the class.

Name of Physician _____

Diagnosis _____

Limitation _____

Areas To Emphasize _____

Medications _____

Physical Activity Profile

Name: _____

Date: _____

We would like to know more about you in order to improve our fitness program and meet your individual needs. Please fill in the following:

1. What was/is the nature of your employment (e.g., manufacturing, sales, teacher)? _____
   Year of retirement, if applicable: _____

2. How would you rate the physical activity you perform/performed at work? (Check one.)
   ____ little (sitting, typing, driving, talking)
   ____ moderate (standing, walking, bending, reaching)
   ____ active (light physical work, climbing stairs)
   ____ very active (moderate and physical work, lifting)

3. My physical activity during the "working hours" of the day has:
   ___ stayed the same   ___ decreased   ___ increased

4. What physical and recreational activities are you presently involved in (e.g., dancing, swimming, walking, bowling)? _____
   _____ How often? _____

5. My goal(s) for joining a fitness program is:
   ___ to lose body fat   ___ to stay active
   ___ because my doctor advised me to   ___ because I am concerned about my health (e.g., blood pressure, arthritis, bad back)

6. Check the activity you participate in and place the appropriate category next to the activity:
   1 if total time spent is less than 15 minutes (3 times/day)
   2 if total time spent is at least 20 minutes (3 times/week)
   3 if activity is sustained for more than 20 minutes (3 times/week)
   ___ walking   ___ swimming   ___ golf
   ___ jogging   ___ dancing   ___ other _____

Appendix 2-H

Medical History Form

Name: _____ Date: _____

1. Have you any medical complaints at present (i.e., lower back pain, arthritis, neck pain, hypertension, diabetes, cardiovascular problems, etc.)? _____
   _____

2. What major illnesses required hospitalization (give dates)? _____
   _____
   _____

3. Smoking status (circle one):

   a. never smoked   b. smoke now   c. smoked in past, not now

4. History of cardiovascular disease:

   NO YES Personal, if so, what _____
   _____

   NO YES Family history, if so, what _____
   _____

   NO YES Other _____
   _____

5. (Muscular history) Present or previous injury?
   a. NO   b. YES
   c. If yes, specify: _____

6. (Bone-joint history) Present or previous bone or joint disease?
   a. NO   b. YES
   c. If yes, specify: _____

7. Check off each of the following ailments that apply to you:

   _____ Frequent dizziness   _____ Hernia   _____ Diabetes
   _____ Physical impairments, if any, specify: _____
   _____

8. On the average, how many times do you visit your physician each year? ____

9. How many times do you take medication each day? _____
   What types of medications are they? _____

10. Do you have any limitations not mentioned previously that will place limita-
    tions on complete participation in the fitness program? _____

Source: The Senior Lifeline Program, University of Southern Maine.

3

Components of a Class

The physical setting is an important consideration for any activity. The wrong physical environment can work against the best of programs, while the right one can enhance all programs. When the program participants are older adults, specific adaptations can be made to create a comfortable, safe, and encouraging environment. If you think that many of these adaptations are simply common sense, you are already on your way toward establishing empathy (i.e., projecting what it would be like to be in another person's shoes).

Empathy is an important quality to develop and maintain when working with diverse groups. Ask yourself questions such as, What will this room look like to an older person? Will noise from the ventilation system compete with my voice or any background music? Is the size of the room adequate for the activities planned? Will the individuals at the back of the room adequately see any audiovisual aids? These are among the basic questions that must be considered in evaluating the physical space allotted to any activity.

Before beginning your program, consider the following: physical space, safety, needs assessment, program development, and leadership skills.

PHYSICAL SPACE

Class leaders are not always in control of which room or corner of a room they are allotted. Before agreeing to use a particular space for your program, make a mental note of the lighting, width of doorways, chairs, tables, outlets, air conditioners or vents, thermostat, color scheme on walls and baseboards, exits, nearest lavatory, and acoustics.

Lighting should be bright. If windows let in natural light to complement synthetic light, consider the glare factor on sunny days; curtains or blinds are a must. Overhead lighting is best. If only table lamps are available, choose the highest wattage on a three-way bulb. For relaxation exercises, consider turning down the lights. Switching the lights off entirely, either to lead relaxation exercises or to view visual aids, is recommended only if a permanent emergency light remains on, however. When no emergency lights are available, consider using night lights, because someone may have to leave the room when the lights are out. It is essential to make certain that the lighting is good for all activities, whether active or passive.

Doorways should be wide enough to accommodate wheelchairs (i.e., thirty-two inches wide). Also, make sure that the lavatories are wheelchair-accessible.

The chairs available should be comfortable and should provide optimum support. Chairs with arms are preferable, although most places have both types of chairs. In this situation, arrange the chairs alternately so that the participants choose their own chairs. Later, if someone with poor balance is constantly missing out on an armed chair, ask someone to switch with that individual.

Always have at least one table available. It does not have to be large, but it can hold items such as cassette players, equipment, tissues, and outer layers of clothing when all else fails.

More than likely, the location of the nearest electrical outlet will dictate where you set up your equipment. If the outlets are embedded in the floor, remember to tape down any wires. If outlets are in the walls, keep the equipment close to the outlets.

Most heating and cooling units are reasonably quiet. In the event that the one in the classroom is not, ask the maintenance department to service it. Competition from "white noise" produced by large units will override any soft voice or music.

Older adults are most comfortable in temperatures that range from seventy-two to seventy-five degrees. Air conditioning can be brutal to an older adult with poor circulation, as can inadequate heating.

Older adults see warm colors, such as reds and oranges, with greater acuity than they see cooler colors, such as blues and greens. When selecting colors for props or equipment, keep this in mind. In addition, since depth perception diminishes with age, walls and baseboards should be differentiated from landings and stairwells by color.

High-frequency hearing loss (presbycusis) is common in older adults, particularly in older men. Therefore, they do not hear high pitches as well as they hear low pitches. Speaking in a well-articulated manner and projecting your voice will help these older adults to hear you.

Avoid competition from a blaring record player or cassette player. Music should enhance your activities, not overwhelm them. Whenever possible, eliminate white noise from any other source. If you are given space in a corner of a large room that is being used simultaneously for other purposes, consider using partitions to block off unwanted noise.

SAFETY

Always think about safety. Look for slippery floors, broken chairs, poor lavatory accessibility, wheelchair accessibility, extension cords untaped on the ground, and poor lighting, to name a few. Also, note the location of fire exits and plan procedures for escape in case of fire prior to the beginning of your program. Note the location of the nearest exit from the building; this exit is also an entrance, should outside help or visitors need access.

NEEDS ASSESSMENT

Although you are ready to conduct a series of health promotion activities, whether they be classes in exercise or in stress management skills, you should poll your participants to determine their ability level, personal interests, and needs. This can be done informally by questioning each individual participant, or it can be done in writing by handing out index cards and asking the participants to respond to a few simple questions. Following are examples of such questions:

- Do you move about without much difficulty?
- Do you have pain in any part of your body when you exercise? If so, where?
- Are you interested in any special topics related to health?

- Do you live alone?
- Are you on any medication? If so, what is the medication for?
- What kinds of health topics interest you?

Not all of these questions are necessary if you are part of a health care team, as the team's access to each participant's medical records will eliminate the need for questions such as the first one.

PROGRAM DEVELOPMENT

No matter how brief or extended, a health promotion program should always have an overall goal with clear objectives. The objectives of your program establish the process by which you do things. Once the process is complete, remember that a follow-up is necessary. Program follow-up can be arranged on the last day of a series by setting a date and time for a return event. Telephone calls, monthly support group meetings, a note in the mail, or a six-month gala event are alternatives.

In developing your program, remember that (1) planning originates in the interests of the participants; (2) objectives are used as the process; (3) participants are encouraged to be leaders; (4) events and progress should be recorded for future use; (5) session evaluations are necessary; and (6) follow-up is a must.

LEADERSHIP SKILLS

Books, manuals, personality tools, and psychological tools have been developed to determine leadership capacity and to train potential leaders. Although a leader is often perceived as someone who is gregarious or highly personable, there is another side of leadership. According to an old Chinese proverb, "A good leader leads his [or her] people into action; a great leader watches as new leaders emerge from his [or her] following."

Qualifications of Class Leaders

Qualified exercise and health education leaders should consider being:

* 1. trained in the areas directly related to physical exercise and aging
  2. skilled in providing a mixture of activities that are purposeful, yet fun
* 3. able to relate meaningfully to the older adult
  4. willing, interested, and empathic
  5. patient (with themselves and others)
  6. organized in their methods and direction
  7. firm, but not authoritarian
* 8. trained in the areas of group dynamics
* 9. trained in basic first aid and cardiopulmonary resuscitation (CPR)
*10. trained to recognize signs of overexertion
  11. certified by the American College of Sports Medicine as a fitness leader, exercise specialist, or exercise test technologist
  12. certified by the National Strength and Conditioning Association

Creativity and the Choice of Music

Another important quality, which may take time to develop, is creativity. Perhaps the most helpful tool in the development of creativity for both leader and participant is music. The right tune can motivate, stimulate, and add new vigor to an old activity, helping the leader and the group to express their creativity.

Songs may be compiled from a number of sources. Libraries and the *Time-Life* record series may be helpful in locating earlier songs. Whatever your choice, do not stereotype the music preferences of older

---

*Essential qualifications

adults. Nostalgia serves its purpose, but a good mix of music with proper tempo and rhythm for a given exercise is the key. Among the appropriate songs are:

- popular songs between 1918 and 1929
    1. *I'm Always Chasing Rainbows*
    2. *K-K-K-Katy*
    3. *Oh, How I Hate To Get up in the Morning*
    4. *Til We Meet Again*
    5. *I'm Forever Blowing Bubbles*
    6. *I'll Be with You in Apple Blossom Time*
    7. *Margie*
    8. *Ain't We Got Fun*
    9. *April Showers*
    10. *I'm Just Wild about Harry*
    11. *Ma, He's Making Eyes at Me*
    12. *Carolina in the Morning*
    13. *Charleston*
    14. *Yes, We Have No Bananas*
    15. *California, Here I Come*
    16. *It Had To Be You*
    17. *Tea for Two*
    18. *Yes, Sir, That's My Baby*
    19. *Birth of the Blues*
    20. *Bye, Bye, Blackbird*
    21. *Sweet Georgia Brown*
    22. *When the Red, Red Robin Comes Bob-Bob-Bobbin' Along*
    23. *Button up Your Overcoat*
    24. *I Can't Give You Anything But Love, Baby*
    25. *Moonlight and Roses*
    26. *Ain't Misbehavin'*
    27. *Happy Days Are Here Again*
    28. *Stardust*
    29. *Singing in the Rain*

- popular songs between 1930 and 1939
    1. *Embraceable You*
    2. *I Got Rhythm*
    3. *On the Sunny Side of the Street*
    4. *Would You Like To Take a Walk?*
    5. *Somebody Loves You*
    6. *Easter Parade*
    7. *Fit as a Fiddle*
    8. *Lazy Bones*
    9. *I Get a Kick out of You*
    10. *The Object of My Affection*
    11. *You Oughta Be in Pictures*
    12. *Begin the Beguine*
    13. *Cheek to Cheek*
    14. *I'm in the Mood for Love*
    15. *It Ain't Necessarily So*
    16. *Goody Goody*
    17. *I've Got You under My Skin*
    18. *Thanks for the Memories*
    19. *Beer Barrel Polka*
    20. *Jeepers Creepers*

- popular songs between 1940 and 1949
    1. *You Must Have Been a Beautiful Baby*
    2. *Chattanooga Choo Choo*
    3. *Don't Sit under the Apple Tree*
    4. *As Time Goes By*
    5. *That Ol' Black Magic*
    6. *Mairzy Doats*
    7. *Buttons and Bows*
    8. *Nature Boy*
    9. *It's a Most Unusual Day*

- popular songs between 1950 and 1959
    1. *If I Knew You Were Coming*
    2. *La Vie en Rose*
    3. *Music, Music, Music*
    4. *My Foolish Heart*
    5. *A Bushel and a Peck*
    6. *Too Young*
    7. *You, You, You*
    8. *Young at Heart*
    9. *Sixteen Tons*
    10. *The Yellow Rose of Texas*
    11. *Hot Diggity*
    12. *Banana Boat Song*
    13. *Chances Are*
    14. *Sugar Time*
    15. *Mack the Knife*
    16. *Smoke Gets in Your Eyes*

- popular songs between 1960 and 1969
    1. *Theme from ''A Summer Place''*
    2. *Roses Are Red*
    3. *The Twist*
    4. *Mashed Potato Time*
    5. *The Stripper*

- popular songs between 1970 and the present
    1. *Fiddler on the Roof*
    2. *Cabaret*
    3. *Hello, Dolly*
    4. *Chanson D'Amour* (Manhattan Transfer)
    5. *Save the Bones for Henry Jones* (Pointer Sisters)
    6. *Shout* (Pointer Sisters)
    7. *Theme from "The Young and the Restless"*
    8. *Don't Worry, Be Happy*

Artists and composers who may offer just the right tempo include

- Michael Jackson (*Off the Wall* and *Thriller* albums)
- George Michaels
- Beach Boys
- Willie Nelson (*Stardust*)
- Mozart
- Strauss
- Chopin
- Ravel

4

The Class Routine

LECTURE/DISCUSSION

Begin each class by introducing yourself and giving a little information about your professional background as it relates to the topic of that day. For example, "Hello, my name is Carole Smith, and I have been a physical therapist for the past ten years. My area of specialty is working with older persons. I received my master's degree in gerontology from the University of Southern California, and I have a private clinic where I see older persons with neurological, musculoskeletal, and cardiopulmonary problems."

In addition, try to personalize any introductory scientific information. If you say something about arthritis, talk about how many people have arthritis. Ask the class participants if they are familiar with physical therapy, if they have ever been to a physical therapist. To learn more about the participants, ask questions such as, What area are you from? How many of you exercise regularly? How many of you go for regular walks? How many of you go to an exercise class? How many of you watch exercise classes on television? You may also want to talk to various class participants about a specific problem as a personal intro-

duction. It is always a nice idea to establish a warm relationship.

Besides general questions, use icebreakers so that you can get to know the class members and they can get to know each other a little better. One good icebreaker is handshaking. Have the participants shake hands with the people next to them. Have them introduce themselves and say hello as a form of an exercise. You can have them do some nodding exercises and say "yes-yes-yes" or "no-no-no" to all of your exercises.

Each class starts with a lecture/discussion. During the lecture, use chalk boards, slides, skeletons, or your body as a visual aid. The more visual aids you use, the more graphic your presentation will be and the more the class participants will remember it. Also, allow time for participants to ask questions. Do not cut them off when they are asking questions, but try to keep individuals from rambling on about their specific problems. If a participant does begin to do that, say that you will talk to him or her after class about the specific problem, but since this is a group, you are going to have to try to answer questions in a more general fashion. This will help keep the group going.

23

WARM UP

Some participants like to do the same warm-up program for every exercise class. They may feel more comfortable with a familiar routine. The warm-up program can be printed on a separate sheet and attached to the printed outline of each exercise program, or it can actually be put on each exercise program as it is designed (Appendix 4-A). The following is a sample outline of a warm-up program that can be adapted to several situations:

1. Deep breaths. Sit back in a chair, get comfortable, and take three nice, deep breaths. (As a variation on the theme, you can ask the participants to make noises as they breathe in or out.) Repeat three times. (See Figure 4-1.)
2. Chin tucks. Gently tuck your chin in and hold it ten seconds. Repeat three times.
3. Shoulder rolls. Roll your shoulders back, then forward three times each.
4. Arm stretchers. Reach your arms straight up in the air as high as you possibly can; reach the right arm over the left and the left arm over the right. Repeat three times.
5. Side reaches. Reach as far as you can to the right and then as far as you can to the left. Repeat three times.
6. Gentle back arches. Gently arch your back with your hands behind your head. Repeat three times.
7. Pelvic tilts. Flatten your back against the chair, and then relax. Repeat three times.
8. Leg strengtheners. Straighten your leg out, and then relax it. Repeat three times. (Your command can be "out and down" three times.)
9. Leg spreads. Spread your legs apart, and bring them together, saying "apart and together." Repeat three times.
10. Ankle bends. Bend each ankle back and forth three times.
11. Toe curls. Curl your toes down and up three times.
12. Ankle circles. Make circles with your ankles in both directions. Repeat three times.

This routine gets the group warmed up before you begin your specific exercise program.

WORK OUT

After several classes, the participants will all know the warm-up routine, but they will not know the specific exercises for a class. Therefore, after the warm-up, go through the new exercises. For example, if the class is about balance, show them how to do the hip circles. Then do the exercise with the group. Finally, repeat the exercise one more time, together. The group actually sees and does the exercise about three times. Once you have gone through the whole program from warm-ups to the exercises, go through the entire exercise program to music.

COOL DOWN

The cool-down session is comprised of some gentle movement and stretching exercises. These let the participants relax and reduce their heart rate and blood pressure so that they do not get up quickly and get dizzy. This gentle session also gives the instructor an opportunity to make sure that everybody is fine after the exercise session. Cool-down exercises are very similar to warm-up exercises, although cool-down exercises are done more slowly and there are not quite as many of them (Appendix 4-A).

A good ending for each exercise session is deep breathing. When doing the final breathing exercise, have the participants visualize their bodies becoming more alert and vital with each breath. You can say, "As you breathe in, feel your body becoming more alert and energetic. Breathe in,

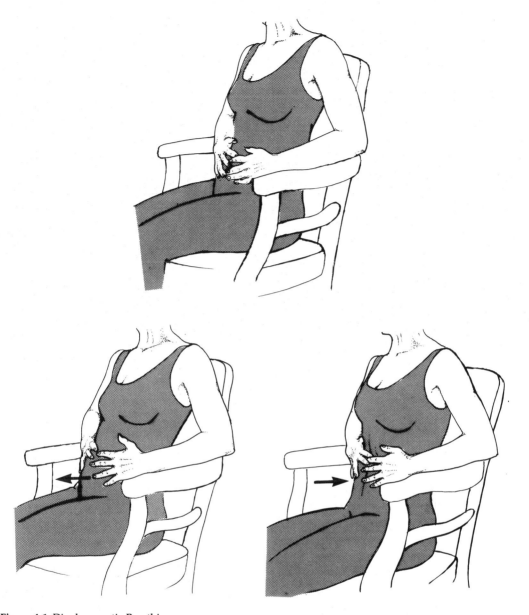

Figure 4-1 Diaphragmatic Breathing

feel the energy, and let out all the bad feelings as you breathe out, and again. . . ."

CONCLUSION

The class routine depends on the creativity of the instructor, the versatility of the group, and the membership of the group. If the participants change at each session, it may be necessary to re-instruct the participants in the warm-ups and cooldowns at each session. If the group remains the same, it may be unnecessary to go over each exercise. Sometimes participants like to change exercise sessions, so you may have to change the warm-ups and cooldowns. The key is to be as motivating and challenging as possible without confusing your exercise participants.

Appendix 4-A

Class Routine Handout

Warm-Up Exercises

1. Deep breaths: Repeat three times.
2. Chin tucks: Repeat three times.
3. Shoulder rolls: Repeat three times each.
4. Arm stretchers: Repeat three times.
5. Side reaches: Repeat three times.
6. Gentle back arches: Repeat three times.
7. Pelvic tilts: Repeat three times.
8. Leg strengtheners: Repeat three times.
9. Leg spreads: Repeat three times.
10. Ankle bends: Repeat three times.
11. Toe curls: Repeat three times.
12. Ankle circles: Repeat three times.

Cool-Down Exercises

1. Ankle bends: Do three times slowly.
2. Ankle circles: Do three times slowly.
3. Leg straighteners: Do three times slowly.
4. Pelvic tilts: Do three times slowly.
5. Shoulder shrugs: Do three times backwards, three times forward.
6. Chin tucks: Do three times.
7. Deep breaths: Do three times.

Part II

Classes

Fancy Footwork

Many problems with walking and balance can be quickly relieved by fixing your feet.

Come to our class and learn more about . . .

FANCY FOOTWORK

at:

_____

on:

_____

in:

_____

Taught by: _____

LISTEN, LEARN, AND EXERCISE!

FANCY FOOTWORK

Health Promotion and Exercise for Older Adults
© Copyright Aspen Publishers, Inc., 1990.
29

5

Fancy Footwork

LECTURE/DISCUSSION

Feet and ankles are amazingly versatile parts of the body. They permit enough motion for us to do many activities, yet they are strong enough to support the entire weight of the body. The foot and ankle are made up of quite a few bones, ligaments, and muscles. For example, the toes are actually a number of bones that are held together by ligaments and are moved by muscles. We have 15 joints in our toe areas, and we have additional joints in the ankle. The ankle joint is called a mortise joint (*show the class what a mortise joint looks like*), which allows the foot to bend forward, backward, and from side to side. These motions are called plantarflexion, dorsiflexion, inversion, and eversion (*show each*). Remember this when we begin to talk about some of the problems of the foot and ankle joints.

Our toes, as you can see, bend in flexion; they also extend (*show the class either on the foot or the hand*). In addition, they abduct (*show the class*). In other words, you are able to spread your toes just like you spread your fingers. However, because our toe muscles are not usually developed to the same degree, this activity may be very difficult.

One very common problem that people have with their feet is the formation of bun-

ions, or hallux valgus. Bunions occur because the big toe is no longer able to move in an appropriate way, and the muscle loses its mechanical advantage because the joint is overstretched to one side. Some people may be generally predisposed to bunions. In the early stages of bunion formation, exercise and positioning can be helpful. After a longer period, however, it is much more difficult to get results with exercise positioning, and surgery may be the only solution.

Another problem that is commonly seen is hammer toes (*show that with your hand*). In this condition, the toes curl upward, again because of some weakness or some malformation in the foot. Poorly fitting shoes contribute to this. A positioning of the back part of the foot and weight bearing on the front part of the foot also add to the problem of hammer toes. Sometimes, orthotics and strengthening exercises can improve hammer toes. As with bunions, however, once a person has had hammer toes for a long time, it is much more difficult to get improvement through orthotics or exercise.

Common problems in the ankle area are sprains or muscle tears. A sprain occurs when the ankle turns out or in and the ligaments that hold the ankle together are slightly torn. There are three types of sprains: mild, moderate, and severe. A mild sprain may be just a pull of the ankle ligaments. A severe sprain is a complete tear in the ligament. In the ankle, stiffness may also be due to arthritis, but this is much less common. The important point to remember about caring for feet and ankles is to keep them moving and strong.

A primary cause of almost all our foot and ankle problems is that we put our feet into shoes that are not correctly fitted. Proper shoe fit should allow a finger's distance between the great toe and the end of the shoe. In addition, when pushing on the sides of the shoe, you should not feel the foot immediately; there should be a slight give before you can feel the foot. If your shoes fit that way, you are probably taking good care of your feet.

Before you leave today, I will give you each a handout with some helpful hints for healthy feet, as well as some do's and don'ts for foot care (*Appendix 5-A; read aloud if you wish*).

Now we are ready to exercise. In performing these exercises, we are going to take it nice and easy with the toes and ankles. These are some very simple exercises, but it is important to do them as slowly as possible and to get a nice, stretching feeling and strengthening while doing them. One fortunate thing about toe and ankle exercises is that they can be done often (e.g., while watching television, talking on the telephone, or working at a desk). So, let us begin.

EXERCISES

1. Toe curls. Curl your toes, and then straighten them. Do this five times.
2. Toe spreads. Spread your toes apart, and bring them together. When doing this, it may help to spread your fingers as you spread your toes. Do this five times.
3. Ankle bends. Bend your ankles up, and then pump them down. Do this four times.

4. Ankle circles. Make a big circle with your ankles in both directions. Do this five times.
5. Toe ups. Put your toes on the ground, and go up on your toes, down, and then up and down again. Repeat five times.
6. Ankle ups. With your feet still on the ground, bend your ankles up and down; lift your toes off the ground, keeping your heels on the ground; just lift your toes up and down. Do this five times.
7. Leg straightening and ankle bends. First, straighten your legs. While your leg is out, bend your ankle up and down. Repeat five times with each leg.
8. Leg straightening and ankle circles. Make big circles with your ankles with your knee in the straightened position. Do these each five times.
9. Towel curls. Crimp a towel up with your toes. Crimp it way up under your toes, and then spread it out with your foot. Repeat five times.
10. Towel slides. Lay a towel sideways, and gently pull the towel across the floor with your foot. Slide the material until no material is left to gather. Do this five times.
11. Foot massage. Rest your foot on your knee, and gently rub the muscles in the bottom of your foot. Give yourself a nice foot massage by rubbing your foot up and down.
12. Toe pulls. *Gently* pull your toes out of the socket and relax. Repeat with each toe. Do this three times.
13. Passive toe bends. Go back to your big toe, and *gently* bend it as far as it will go forward. Hold ten seconds, and then release. Bend the next toe as far as it will go, hold 10 seconds, and release. Do this to all your toes.

(*Go down the list of exercises and back with the music, repeating instructions as necessary. At the end, tell the participants to use their handout and do the exercises daily at home.*)

Appendix 5-A

Fancy Footwork Handout

Hints

1. Try to avoid wearing shoes that are too small.
2. Try to elevate your feet as often as you can.
3. Move your toes around as much as possible.

Do's

1. Keep your feet warm.
2. Watch for cuts and bruises on your feet.
3. Do toe and ankle exercises regularly.
4. Try to buy high-quality shoes.
5. Make sure you have a finger's width of room from the end of your longest toe to your shoe.

Don'ts

1. Do not wear tight-fitting shoes.
2. Do not wear clothes that are too tight in the leg area.
3. Do not sit with your feet in the dependent position for a long period of time.

4. Do not expose your feet to the cold.
5. Do not wear socks that are worn out, excessively wrinkled, or dirty, or shoes that are improperly fitted.

Exercises

1. Toe curls: Do this five times.
2. Toe spreads: Do this five times.
3. Ankle bends: Do this four times.
4. Ankle circles: Do this five times.
5. Toe ups: Repeat five times.
6. Ankle ups: Do this five times.
7. Leg straightening and ankle bends: Repeat five times with each leg.
8. Leg straightening and ankle circles: Repeat five times with each leg.
9. Towel curls: Repeat five times.
10. Towel slides: Do this five times.
11. Foot massage: Repeat five times.
12. Toe pulls: Do this three times.
13. Passive toe bends: Do this to all your toes.

Lavish Legs

Learn the secrets of Fred Astaire and Ginger Rogers . . . . What muscles and bones made their legs so graceful and agile. . . .

This class will explain the workings of the legs, as well as common leg problems.

LAVISH LEGS

at:

_____

on:

_____

in:

_____

Taught by: _____

LISTEN, LEARN, AND EXERCISE!

LAVISH LEGS

6

Lavish Legs

LECTURE/DISCUSSION

Legs can take us any place we want to go; help us to imitate Fred Astaire, Ginger Rogers, or the Rockettes; and allow us to go up and down stairs. What happens to our legs as we get older? Normally, there is a decrease in muscle mass (atrophy) after age 30 due to a decrease in the number and the size of the muscle fibers in the legs. Because muscle cells do not regenerate, it is very important to keep the remaining muscle tissues strong and flexible. If muscles are not stretched and trained routinely for strength and joint integrity, weakness sets in.

Muscle weakness can be caused by poor nutrition, lack of sufficient nerve stimulation, illness, loss of muscle tissue, or disuse. Although we cannot reverse a weakness related to chronic disease or aging, we can somewhat right the effects of weakness related to disuse.

In order to exercise our legs effectively, it may help to know what specific bones and muscles do. Muscles are interesting. They are arranged in pairs so that, as one contracts, the other lengthens; this creates a smooth and controlled movement. The gentle, constant pulling of muscles against each other gives the body muscle tone.

Basically, there are three types of muscles: skeletal, as in the legs; cardiac, located only in the heart; and smooth, as in the intestines. Skeletal muscles contract and relax quickly, but they can also tire quickly. That is one reason that it is important to use them efficiently and effectively.

Muscles have different parts to them. The muscle belly, which is the fleshier part of the muscle, slims down to form a tendon, which attaches the muscle to the bone.

There are several muscles to keep toned in the legs. For example, the quadriceps (*show where*) are the muscles that extend the leg. The opposite action is done by the hamstrings (*show them*). This group of muscles goes from the hip to the rear of the knee (*show them*). There is another large group of muscles that most of us are quite aware of: the gluteals. The largest of these is the gluteus maximus (*show them*), which extends (*demonstrate*), abducts (*demonstrate*), and rotates (*demonstrate*) the hip to the side.

The bones in the leg include the femur, which is the longest, largest, and heaviest bone in the body. The femur extends from the pelvis to the knee. The shin bone, or tibia, is the larger of the two bones in the lower leg. The fibula, the second bone in the lower leg, runs alongside the tibia and touches it at this point (*show approximate location*).

Before we begin to exercise, we should talk about various conditions of the leg. Some of us have occasional or constant pain from varicose veins, a hereditary condition in which enlarged veins appear very close to the skin's surface. They are easily spotted as dark blue lines on the leg, often extending up and down for several inches. They appear because the valves inside the blood vessels, which are supposed to keep blood moving toward the heart, are malfunctioning. Therefore, the pull of gravity keeps the blood in the legs. This pooled blood distends and enlarges the veins. Sometimes clots form in varicose veins. A vein with a clot in it is red and swollen, and it hurts when touched. If this happens to you, do not do any exercises or vigorous activity, and see your doctor.

Support hose may alleviate some of the pain from varicose veins, as does sitting with your legs uncrossed. Never stand in one place for a prolonged period either. Exercise can help treat varicose veins as long as you exercise daily.

Occluded or clogged arteries in the leg are often "silent." Usually, 80 percent of all arteries are occluded before there is any pain. This condition may be called peripheral arterial disease. A major symptom is pain in the legs after exercising or walking. Eating fried or fatty foods and smoking are risk factors that may contribute to such a condition. Exercising regularly, eating a proper diet, quitting smoking, and taking medication, if necessary, will help control the pain.

The last condition we are going to talk about is pain in the legs at night, a frequent complaint of both older and younger adults. Sometimes it is a sign of fatigue, a result of muscle weakness after a day of excessive walking, or a symptom of arthritis. Exercising and putting your feet up on pillows in bed are two ways to increase the circulation and control the pain. Also, massage your legs in a motion toward your heart, not down toward your feet. Let's try

this together before we review some do's and don'ts for your legs (*show the class how to massage the legs*). I'll give you a handout with some suggestions on ways to keep your legs healthy before you leave (*Appendix 6-A; read aloud if you wish*).

EXERCISES

1. Postural awareness. Sit up straight with both feet firmly planted on the floor, arms relaxed, and hands gently sitting in your lap. Wriggle your toes, and feel your feet planted firmly on the floor as you adjust your posture to support your lower back.
2. Single leg swing. Clasp your hands under your right knee. Elevate your leg slowly off the chair, and swing your leg forward and back for ten full swings. Repeat with the left leg.
3. Bent single leg raises. Inhale normally, and, as you exhale, lift up your right leg. Repeat four more times. Follow the same directions for your left leg.
4. Outer leg presses. Place the palms of the hands flat against the outside of the knees. Using your palms as resistance, push your knees against them. Remember to breathe out as you push in. Never hold your breath. Repeat four more times.
5. Inner leg presses. Place the palms of the hands flat against the inside of the knees. Using your palms as resistance, push against your knees. Breathe out as you push. Repeat the exercise four more times. Breathe normally in the relaxed position between exercises.
6. Leg raises. Raise your right leg with the knee slightly bent, and hold the position as the knee joint straightens out the lower leg. Slowly and gently, lift the entire leg no more than an inch off the chair. Keep the left leg relaxed with the left foot flat on the ground. Clasping your hands onto

each side of the chair will help you to balance. Repeat twice more. Repeat with your left leg.

7. Double leg raises. This exercise is hard. Start slowly and don't hold your breath at any point during this exercise. Place your hands at each side of the chair, and grasp the underside. Slide your bottom toward the front of the chair, making sure that you remain comfortable and are not about to fall or slide off your chair. Inhale deeply, and, on exhaling, raise both legs off the ground. Hold that position for a count of five, but do not hold your breath at any time.

8. Fake tippy toes. As you remain seated, starting with your feet together, use the balls of your feet to step with, taking each foot past the corner of each chair. This is done quickly, as the legs are brought apart and then together. Repeat five times.

9. Beanbag flip. Place a beanbag on the tip of your right foot. Aim the beanbag at the wastebasket placed in the center of the exercisers' circle and try to flip it in. Place a second beanbag on your left foot. Try to flip it into the same wastebasket. Now, get up out of your chair to retrieve your beanbags. Walk back to your chair. Place the beanbags under your chair, and stand behind your chair.

10. Calf stretches. Holding onto your chair, place both feet together. Now raise up on your toes, and hold that position for a count of five. Return to a relaxed position, and then repeat for another count of five.

11. Side lifts. Walk to the right side of your chair. Holding on with your left hand, face the front of the chair, making sure that your pelvis is straight. Now, slowly raise your right leg sideways to a comfortable position, and hold the position for a count of five. Return to the center position. Repeat five times. Repeat the entire exercise using your left leg.

12. Back kicks. Stand behind your chair, positioning yourself at the center of the chair. Place both hands on the chair back. Without leaning too far forward, raise the right leg back. If you feel any pain in your lower back, relax the leg until you no longer feel it, and continue the exercise to that point only. Do not tilt forward. Return to center position. Repeat five times. Repeat entire exercise with left leg.

13. Small knee bends. Stand behind your chair. Bend your knees halfway while holding your arms out in front of you holding the chair back, palms facing down (Figure 6-1). Hold for a second, making sure your heels are flat against the floor. Return to starting position. Repeat five times.

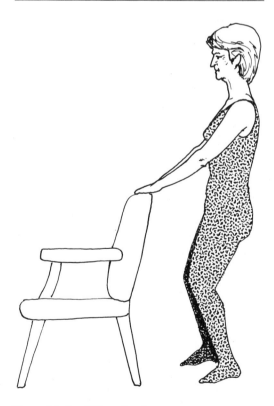

Figure 6-1 Small Knee Bends

14. Classic stork stand (use partners or chairs for balance, if needed). Stand tall with your feet slightly apart. Place your hands on your hips, holding your head upright. Now, transfer your weight onto your left foot, and bend your right knee. Bring the underside of your right foot to the inside of your left leg, preferably at the knee (Figure 6-2). While extending your arms out to the side for balance, hold this position for about ten seconds. Relax, then repeat with the right leg. When you feel confident about this exercise, progress to stance 3 of Figure 6-2.

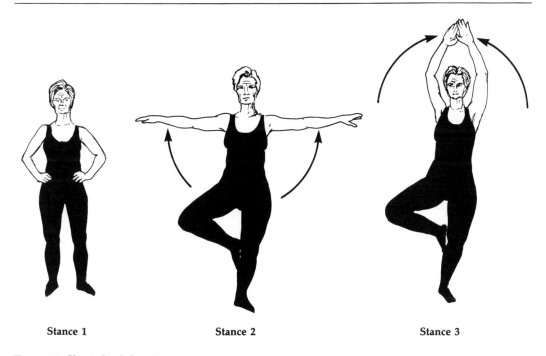

Stance 1   Stance 2   Stance 3

Figure 6-2 Classic Stork Stand

Appendix 6-A

Lavish Legs Handout

Do's

1. Put your feet up for a few minutes each day, or prop your feet up on pillows in bed at night.
2. Stretch your legs every day, slowly and gently.
3. Wear support hose on achy days. They will help to control the pain.
4. Walk up and down hallways or around your room or apartment as much as possible during rainy or snowy days.

Don'ts

1. Do not sit with your legs crossed for any length of time. Doing so cuts off circulation to the legs and feet and makes varicose veins worse.
2. Do not sit or stand in one place for too long. Not only will you feel tired, but also you will allow blood to pool in your legs.
3. Do not wear support hose to exercise. They interfere with the natural cooling mechanism in your body. If you are prevented from sweating, you will tire more easily when exercising.

Exercises

1. Postural awareness.
2. Single leg swing: Repeat five times with each leg.
3. Bent single leg raises: Repeat five times with each leg.
4. Outer leg presses: Repeat five times.
5. Inner leg presses: Repeat five times.
6. Leg raises: Repeat five times.
7. Double leg raises: Repeat five times.
8. Fake tippy toes: Repeat five times.
9. Beanbag flip: Repeat five times.
10. Calf stretches: Repeat five times.
11. Side lifts: Repeat five times.
12. Back kicks: Repeat five times.
13. Small knee bends: Repeat five times.
14. Classic stork stand: Repeat five times.

Knowledgeable Knees

Learn about one of the most unstable yet hard-working joints in the body . . .

KNOWLEDGEABLE KNEES

at:

_____

on:

_____

in:

_____

Taught by: _____

LISTEN, LEARN, AND EXERCISE!

KNOWLEDGEABLE KNEES

Knowledgeable Knees

LECTURE/DISCUSSION

Although the knee joint may look like a simple joint, it is one of the most complex. Moreover, the knee is more likely to be injured than is any other joint in the body. We tend to ignore our knees until something happens to them that causes some pain. As the saying goes, however, "an ounce of prevention is worth a pound of cure." If we take good care of our knees now, before there is a problem, we can really help ourselves. In addition, if some problems with the knees develop, an exercise program can be extremely beneficial.

The knee is essentially made up of four bones. The femur, which is the large bone in your thigh (*show the class*), attaches by ligaments in a capsule to your tibia (*show the class*). Just below the tibia is the fibula, which runs parallel to the tibia. The patella, or what we call the knee cap, rides on the knee joint as the knee bends (*have a picture or a model to help demonstrate the anatomy*).

When the knee moves, it does not just bend and straighten, or, as it is medically termed, flex and extend. There is also a slight rotation component in this motion. This component was recognized only within the last 50 years, which may be part of the reason why people have so many unknown injuries. The knee muscles that cross the knee joint are the quadriceps (*show them*) and the hamstrings (*show them*); quadriceps are on the front of the knee, and hamstrings are on the back of the knee. The ligaments are equally important in the knee joint because they hold the joint together. You may have heard of people who have had ligament tears or ligament surgeries. Problems with ligaments are common (*show the position of the cruciate ligaments and the collateral ligaments*). In review, the bones support the knee and provide the rigid structure of the joint, the muscles move the joint, and the ligaments stabilize the joint.

The knee joint also has a structure made of cartilage, which is called the meniscus. The cartilage protects the joint and allows the bones to slide freely on each other (*demonstrate with your fists where the cartilage is in the knee*). There is also a bursa around the knee joint. A bursa is a little fluid sac that helps the muscles and tendons slide freely as the knee moves.

To function well, a person needs to have strong and flexible muscles; the cartilage, ligaments, and bursa must be smooth and strong as well. Problems occur when any of these parts of the knee joint are irritated.

One problem is tendinitis, which is an inflammation of the tendons connecting the muscles and the knee. Bursitis, an inflammation of the bursa, can occur from overuse, such as repeated bending or leaning weight on the knee. Kneeling on the knee cap causes pressure on the bursa and may cause significant pain (*show where this is*).

Arthritis is a common disease that affects the knee and is characterized by degeneration of the cartilage, causing pain and swelling. Many people believe that overuse of a knee joint can cause arthritis, even though there has been no definitive research to confirm this belief. There are also malalignment problems with knees, such as bow legs, knock knees, and back knees. Any of these positions can cause undue stress and weight bearing to the knee, which could eventually lead to arthritis.

Appropriate and slow exercise can help knee problems, but it is extremely important not to do anything that causes your knee pain. Consider slowly increasing the intensity of your program when exercising to make your knees feel better.

Before the class is over today, I will give each of you a handout with some dos and don'ts for healthy knees (*Appendix 7-A, read aloud if desired*).

EXERCISES

Sitting

1. Knee bends. Bend each knee three times.
2. Quad sets.
   (a) Tighten the muscles on top of the thigh as tightly as possible and hold. It will help with this and other exercises if, while you tighten, you pull your toes back toward your face, push the back of your knee down to the floor, and try to push out and up through the heel.

(b) Hold ten seconds, trying every second to hold even tighter. Relax five seconds. Repeat ten times. Rest 20 seconds between sets.
3. Static leg holds. Keeping the knee bent, place a hard object under the leg to hold it at a height of about six inches. Raise the lower leg until your knee is as straight as possible, and do a quad set. Again, pull the toes back, push down on the block, push out and up through the heel. Pull ten seconds, trying every second to hold tighter. Relax five seconds. Repeat ten times, resting between sets. Rest 20 seconds.
4. Straight leg raises. (Do not do this exercise if you have hip pain.) Tighten the muscles on the top of your thigh as tightly as possible and hold for entire exercise. Try and pull even tighter. Keeping *all* of this tension, raise the entire leg four inches. Try again to pull even tighter. Keeping *all* of the tension, lower the leg back to the floor. Try again to pull even tighter. Relax (finally). This is an easy exercise if you concentrate. If you do not tighten the knee muscles to their absolute maximum, you are not gaining much benefit from the straight leg raises. If you have trouble, just stop and rest a moment, after giving it one more try with more concentration. Then continue. Repeat ten times, resting 60 seconds between sets. Rest 20 seconds.
5. Knee bends. Bend each knee three times.
6. Leg spreads. Straighten your knees, and spread your legs apart; then bring them back together. Repeat five times. Arm movements may be added to enhance this exercise (Figure 7-1).
7. Pes pushes. Put your feet together, and keep your knees apart. Gently squeeze your feet against each other. Hold ten seconds. Repeat five times.

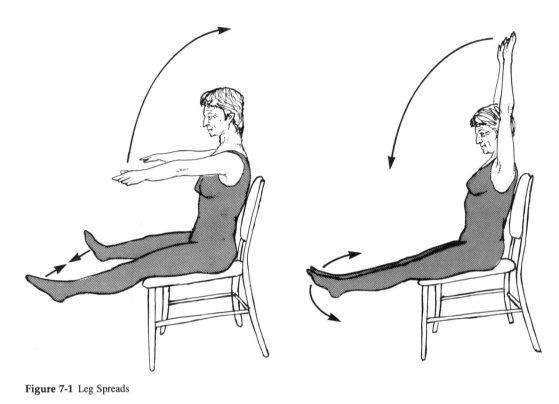

Figure 7-1 Leg Spreads

Standing (While Holding on to a Stable Chair or Counter Top)

8. Toe raises. While standing up straight with your feet together, turn your heels out slightly so that you are now standing a bit "pigeon-toed." Now, raise up and down on your tip toes, making sure to go both ways as far as possible. Try and keep your weight distributed equally on both legs. Repeat 20 times.
9. Heel stretches. Lean forward (holding on to a chair and keeping your heels down) until you feel a stretch in your calves. Hold 20 seconds. Repeat five times.
10. Slight bends. Holding on to a chair, slightly bend your knees and come up. Repeat ten times.
11. Side kicks. Kick your leg sideways. Repeat ten times with each leg.
12. Back kicks. Slowly (move) kick your leg backward. Repeat ten times with each leg.
13. Front kicks. Slowly (move) kick your leg forward. Repeat ten times with each leg.
14. Leg wiggles. Stand on one leg, and shake out the other. Do five times with each leg.

Appendix 7-A

Knowledgeable Knees Handout

Hints

1. A correctly applied knee wrap can be helpful for knee problems because it keeps in the body's heat. It must not be too tight, however.
2. Whenever you have pain in your knee, try to put ice on your knee for 10 to 20 minutes to reduce inflammation.
3. Warm your knees up prior to doing activities, either by applying heat or by gently bending your knees back and forth.
4. If pain persists, contact a physician or physical therapist.

Do's

1. Swim.
2. Sleep on your side with a pillow between your knees.
3. Exercise regularly (unless your knees hurt while you do or for an hour afterward).
4. Bend your knee as often as possible to discourage stiffness and keep the joint in good shape.

5. Wear comfortable shoes and socks.
6. Smile!

Don'ts

1. Do not kneel if it hurts.
2. Do not climb stairs if you don't have to, especially leading with your bad leg.
3. Do not keep walking when your knee hurts.
4. Do not keep your leg in one position too long.
5. Do not do deep knee bends.
6. Do not run or ride a bike with resistance.

Exercises

Sitting

1. Knee bends: Repeat three times.
2. Quad sets: Repeat ten times.
3. Static leg holds: Repeat ten times.
4. Straight leg raises: Repeat ten times.
5. Leg spreads: Repeat five times.

6. Pes pushes: Repeat five times.
7. Knee bends: Repeat three times.

Standing

8. Toe raises: Repeat 20 times.

9. Heel stretches: Repeat five times.
10. Slight bends: Repeat five times.
11. Side kicks: Repeat ten times.
12. Back kicks: Repeat ten times.
13. Front kicks: Repeat ten times.
14. Leg wiggles: Repeat five times.

Happy Hips

When was the last time you had "happy hips"?

The goal of this class is to gain an appreciation of how our hip joints work.

HAPPY HIPS

at:

_____

on:

_____

in:

_____

Taught by: _____

LISTEN, LEARN, AND EXERCISE!

HAPPY HIPS

Happy Hips

LECTURE/DISCUSSION

The hip is one of the most stable joints in the body. Because of its function in bearing the body's weight, however, it may be susceptible to arthritis due to excessive pressure. The hip joint is a ball and socket joint. The socket area, which is inside your pelvis, is called the acetabulum (*indicate the area*). The ball part of this joint is the top of the leg bone. It joins with the acetabulum to form the hip joint. These are actually held together by ligaments, muscles, and the joint capsule. This arrangement allows motion, yet provides the stability needed to bear all the rest of your body weight on your legs.

The structures in the hip joint are the capsule, which is a tough, stretchy material; the ligaments, which go all the way around and outside this capsule; and the muscles, which are attached by tendons and are all around the hip joint. Some of the muscles that go around your hip are your hip flexors, which flex your hips (*demonstrate*); your hip abductors, which bring your leg out to the side (*show the group where these muscles [e.g., the gluteus medius and the tensor fascia lata] are*); and the hip extensors,

which bring your leg back. In addition, the hip also rotates internally and externally (*demonstrate hip rotation*). Internal rotators such as abductors (*indicate the area*) turn the legs in, and external rotators turn the legs out. These are tiny little muscles on the back part of your hip. Because some of the muscles are tiny, they become tighter more easily and can be overpowered by the larger muscles. Therefore, it is important to have a good range of motion that will allow the hip to move freely without pains and strains.

There are two kinds of arthritis that affect the hip. One is osteoarthritis, which is a degeneration of the top of the acetabulum (*indicate the area of the acetabulum*) because of the constant weight bearing there. The other is rheumatoid arthritis, which is a wearing inside. Many times surgery, medication, and progressive non–weight-bearing exercises are needed for these problems. It is very important to avoid lifting the whole leg in hip exercises, however, because this could cause excessive stress on the hip joint.

Another problem associated with the hips is bursitis, a condition in which the little sacs around the muscles become inflamed because the muscles are taking on too much stress. Whenever you feel pain in your hip from arthritis or bursitis, it is a good idea to slow down what you are doing; cut the activity in half until the pain goes away, and then increase the activity again as you feel better.

I will give each of you a handout with hints to keep your hips healthy (*Appendix 8-A; read aloud if desired*).

EXERCISES

Sitting

1. Knee to chest exercises. Pull *one* knee toward your chest gently, without causing pain, and put it back down (Figure 8-1). Repeat ten times.
2. Seat lifts. Gently lift your seat off the chair, and then put it back down. Repeat ten times.
3. Leg spreads. Spread your legs apart, and then place them together. Repeat ten times.
4. Leg rolls. Straighten your legs, roll your legs out, and then roll your legs in. Repeat ten times.
5. Knee bend twists. Bend your knee, and then pull your ankle up. Then pull your ankle out to the side. Repeat five times.
6. Hip rocks. Rock your hips forward and backward in the chair. Repeat ten times.
7. Moshe (named after Moshe Feldenkrais): Gently put your hands on your knees, and gently move your legs forward and backward, one at a time from the hips. Repeat ten times.

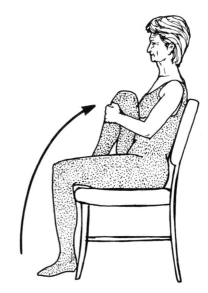

Figure 8-1 Knee to Chest Exercise

8. Hip circles. Make a big circle in your chair with your hips in both directions. Repeat ten times.

Standing (While Holding on to a Stable Chair or Countertop)

9. Backward leg kicks. Kick your leg backwards. Repeat ten times.
10. Side kicks. Kick your leg out to the side. Repeat ten times.
11. Leg ins. Pull your leg in toward the other leg, and cross it over at the ankles. Repeat ten times.
12. March in place. Pull your legs up as high as you can and march in place. Repeat ten times.
13. Honolulu roll. Make big circles with your hips in each direction. Repeat ten times.

Appendix 8-A

Happy Hips Handout

Hints

1. Sleep on your side with a pillow between your knees.
2. Put ice on sore areas of the hip as often as possible.
3. Avoid lifting your leg straight in the air. Try to bend your knee and use your hand to help you.

Do's

1. Exercise as often as possible.
2. Sit and sleep in comfortable positions.
3. Massage your muscles in the hip area when they are sore.

Don'ts

1. Do not sleep on the painful side of your hip.
2. Do not stand in painful positions.

3. Do not continue with activities that cause pain.

Exercises

Sitting

1. Knee to chest exercises: Repeat ten times.
2. Seat lifts: Repeat ten times.
3. Leg spreads: Repeat ten times.
4. Leg rolls: Repeat ten times.
5. Knee bend twists: Repeat five times.
6. Hip rocks: Repeat ten times.
7. Moshe: Repeat ten times.
8. Hip circles: Repeat ten times.

Standing

9. Back leg kicks: Repeat ten times.
10. Side kicks: Repeat ten times.
11. Leg ins: Repeat ten times.
12. March in place: Repeat ten times.
13. Honolulu rolls: Repeat ten times.

Better Backs

Oh, my aching back! Have you ever said this to yourself? If so, you should attend the Better Backs class.

We will explore different ways of strengthening and improving your back. You will receive extremely helpful hints and exercises.

BETTER BACKS

at:

_____

on:

_____

in:

_____

Taught by: _____

LISTEN, LEARN, AND EXERCISE!

BETTER BACKS

9

Better Backs

LECTURE/DISCUSSION

The back is one of the most complex, most studied, and most misunderstood areas of the body. The back, or spinal column, is made up of small segments called vertebrae. These vertebrae are separated by discs, which are little spongy structures that are shaped like a rounded version of an orange section. As we get older, the discs tend to change a bit. The covering of the disc tends to get more fibrous. In addition, the gel-like substance inside of the disc tends to dehydrate as we get older, so that it becomes somewhat thicker. These changes make the disc less pliable.

Muscles are attached to each segment of the spine (*hold up a model of the spine and show where all of the erector spinae attach*). These are tiny little muscles that attach to each segment of the vertebral bodies. Remember that these muscles are very small, because their size will be important later when we talk about lifting and when we talk about the motion of the vertebrae.

There are also small ligaments in the back that, like little rubber bands, hold these vertebral segments together when, for example, the muscles cannot do their job or do not do their job. You may have heard of people who sprain ligaments. This happens in the back, as well as in other joints of the body.

Take a look at what the back can do. You can flex your back, extend it, flex it laterally, and rotate it (*demonstrate each*). Because all of these motions occur in the back region, the vertebrae, muscles, and ligaments have to be supple and strong. Problems occur when the muscles in the back are shortened, tightened, or weakened. A tightening of a muscle is called a muscle spasm or a muscle strain. A tear or a rupture, or just slight damage to the ligaments, is called a ligament sprain. In addition, the disc can rupture so that its contents actually protrude from its covering and put pressure on the nerves that come out of the spine. This condition, sometimes called a herniated disc, can cause some difficulty and severe pain. Discs tend not to rupture as much in older people because there is not as much fluid inside to cause rupture. Nevertheless, older people do occasionally have some problems with this.

Earlier, we talked about the small muscles. Think about the activities you do each day. For example, when you bend over to lift something, you are using the small back muscles. A better way to lift is to squat and use the long muscles on the front of your leg (*demonstrate this*). The bigger muscles can generate more force to lift your body than the smaller muscles of your back can. Many people have accidents when they try to use their shorter muscles to do an activity that they should use their bigger muscles to do (*show the difference between lifting with the legs and lifting with the back*).

The structure of your back may give you some information about injury potential. When you look at your back for structure characteristics, look to see if you are more prone to flattening out or curving in your lower back area. If your back tends to flatten out, you may have more problems with overstretching of the muscles. If your back tends to curve in, you may be more likely to have problems with muscle spasm. So what I want you to do right now is to put your hand on your lower back and see if you would consider your back flat or if you consider your back curved, which is what some people call sway back. An even better way to check this is to do it when standing up (*walk around the room and see if, in fact, the class members have a feel for whose back is flat and whose back is rounded*). Those of you who have a flat back tend to need a little more support in your lower back while you are sitting. Those of you with a curved back, or sway back, generally get more spasms and find it difficult to stand for long periods of time because those muscles work overtime to hold you up. Take breaks and sit for a while to break up long standing sessions. Additional hints for those with curved backs or sway backs are to do more pelvic tilts or flattening (*demonstrate*). Those of you with arched backs and flat backs may want to do more arching (*demonstrate*).

Before you leave today, I will give you a handout with helpful hints on ways to keep your back in good condition (*Appendix 9-A; read aloud if you wish*).

Now, we are going to do some exercises. First, I will show you the exercise. Then, you will do them with me. Then, we will go through them together with music.

EXERCISES

1. Deep breaths. Take three deep breaths.
2. Back relaxers. Take a deep breath in. Bring your hands along your body. Reach toward the ceiling, and, as you bring your hands down to your sides, let all of the muscles relax as your hands pass by. Repeat three times.
3. Pelvic tilts. Flatten your lower back against the back of the chair. Hold it for ten seconds and relax. Repeat three times.
4. Back arches. Gently arch your back. Put your hands in the small of your back, and arch your back. Hold it there for three seconds; then relax. Repeat three times.
5. Back rotators. Slowly turn your trunk to the right, turn to the middle, turn your trunk to the left. Relax. Repeat three times.
6. Side tilts. Hang your right arm over the side of a chair, and tilt to your right. Repeat to the left side. Repeat five times.
7. Moshe. Gently put your hands on your thighs, and gently move your thighs forward and backward, one at a time from the hips. Repeat five times.
8. Knee to chest exercises. In your chair, gently try to bring your knee toward your chest, and put it back down. Repeat three times with each leg.
9. Back hangs. Do not do this exercise if you have osteoporosis or chronic vertigo. Gently hang your body over your knees and let all of the muscles of your back relax. Hold that position for four seconds, and then come back up. Repeat three times.
10. Side reaches. Put your arms out to your side at a 90-degree angle. Reach to your right as far as you can, and come back to the middle. Reach to

your left as far as you can, and come back to the middle. Repeat three times.

11. Forward crossover reaches. With your left arm, reach to the right side as far as you can; then with your right arm, reach to the left side as far as you can. Repeat three times.

12. Head bends. Bend your head forward, and then come back up to the starting position. Repeat three times.

13. Head tilts. Tilt your head to the left, and then come back up. Tilt your head to the right, and come up. Repeat three times.

14. Bottom tighteners. Pinch your bottom together as tight as you can for ten seconds, and then relax. Pinch again, and then relax. Repeat three times, and relax.

The most important thing to remember about back exercises is that they should be done at least once a day. You should be relaxed when you do them. Try not to strain. If the exercises cause any pain, stop them immediately, and consult your physical therapist or physician.

Appendix 9-A

Better Backs Handout

Hints

1. Rest your back whenever you are tired by lying down or sitting comfortably in a supportive chair.
2. Take a warm shower or apply heat to your back before exercise to warm up your back muscles and allow them to stretch better.
3. If you wake up feeling sore in the morning, it usually means that you were sleeping in a position that irritated your back. One way to resolve this problem is simply to experiment with different positions until you wake up pain-free.
4. For those with curved backs, make sure that your knees are higher than your hips to support your back when you sit.

Do's

1. Move around frequently to keep the muscles supple.
2. Support your back in any position that you are in, whether sitting or standing. When sitting, especially during long car rides, put a small pillow behind the lower back and see if that feels more comfortable.
3. Always sit in a good chair that provides support with your feet flat on the floor.
4. Always sleep in a comfortable position. This may mean on your side, curled up in a fetal position, with pillows behind your back or under your knees.
5. Bend with your knees to lift anything.
6. Avoid twisting or jerky movements.

Don'ts

1. Do not bend from the waist to lift heavy things.
2. Do not sit in one position too long.
3. Do not reach over your head for heavy objects, as this movement can put too much stress on the back.

4. Do not stand with poor posture.
5. Do not sleep in soft beds or chairs.

Exercises

1. Deep breaths: Take three deep breaths.
2. Back relaxers: Repeat three times.
3. Pelvic tilts: Repeat three times.
4. Back arches: Repeat three times.
5. Back rotators: Repeat three times.
6. Side tilts: Repeat five times to each side.
7. Moshe: Repeat five times.
8. Knee to chest exercises: Repeat three times with each leg.
9. Back hangs: Repeat three times.
10. Side reaches: Repeat three times to each side.
11. Forward crossover reaches: Repeat three times to each side.
12. Head bends: Repeat three times.
13. Head tilts: Repeat three times to each side.
14. Bottom tighteners: Repeat three times, and relax.

Nice Necks

Don't have a pain in the neck, learn how to prevent one.

Also learn ways of strengthening neck muscles properly and ways to modify your daily activities to decrease neck pain.

NICE NECKS

at:

_____

on:

_____

in:

_____

Taught by: _____

LISTEN, LEARN, AND EXERCISE!

NICE NECKS

10

Nice Necks

LECTURE/DISCUSSION

To begin, put your hands on your necks. What do you feel? You feel skin, muscle, and bone. The neck has an important job—holding up the head. Think about it for a second. Imagine holding a bowling ball in your hand with your arm out to the side. Then imagine holding the bowling ball straight over your head. Which do you think would be easier? Actually, it would be easier to hold the bowling ball over your head, because the weight would be evenly distributed over your body. If you hold the bowling ball out to your side, it becomes very heavy, and, after a few seconds, you may not be able to hold it there any longer. Many people develop neck problems through a similar process. Look at my head in relation to my body in an everyday situation, such as watching television, driving a car, sitting at a desk, and knitting (*demonstrate a forward head position*). This is very much like holding a bowling ball out to the side, rather than over the shoulders. If I could move my neck into a better position so that my head is over my shoulders, I would be putting less stress on the neck muscles, and they would not be working so hard.

In the neck area, there are seven vertebrae, or spinal segments, each separated by discs. These spongy discs, which are much like sections of an orange, allow the head to move easily from one position to another. The muscles direct the movement by moving the head forward, backward, or side to side and rotating the head around its axis. In addition, tiny ligaments, like rubber bands, hold each segment together so that, even if the muscles do not work quickly or effectively, your head remains on your shoulders. The coordination of the muscles, ligaments, and bones determines the efficiency of the neck.

You can move your head forward (*ask the group to do these activities with you*), backward, and side to side; you can turn your head to look over your shoulders. Let me show you what full motion is. Full forward motion is bringing your chin all the way down to your chest. Full extension is bringing the back of your head to rest on your back (*before you demonstrate full extension, you may want to tell the group not to do this if it hurts or if they get dizzy*). Full lateral flexion is bringing your head to a point about halfway between your shoulder and the starting position, which is head tilting. Full rotation is looking over your shoulder with your chin evenly over that shoulder. Some of you are noticing that you are a little limited there. That is nothing to worry about unless it causes pain.

The exercises that we are going to do today will help to loosen your neck muscles. If we do not stretch these muscles to the limit, the muscles will get shorter. If we spend most of the day with the neck in one position, that is what happens. The following exercises are designed to get you to use the muscles in your neck as often as possible so that they do not become tight and painful. After we exercise, I will give you a sheet with helpful hints to keep your neck healthy (*Appendix 10-A; read aloud and discuss if you wish*). All right, it is time to begin our exercises. We are going to slowly go through these exercises, beginning with deep breaths and then going to the arm reaches and shoulder shrugs, and then we will return to deep breaths.

EXERCISES

1. Deep breaths. Begin with three deep breaths. Take a deep breath in, and exhale as much as possible. Repeat three times.
2. Shoulder shrugs. Roll your shoulders back, and then roll them forward. Repeat five times.
3. Head bends. Bend head forward and back. Remember, if the back position hurts you, *stop immediately*. Repeat five times.
4. Head turns. Turn your head, and look over your shoulder. Repeat five times.
5. Head tilts. Bring your ear toward your shoulder as far as you can. If it hurts on the same side, however, you should stop. If you get a little pain or stretch on the opposite side, that is okay, but do not overdo. It should feel only a little stretched, not painful. Repeat five times.
6. Arm clasp reaches. Clasp your hands, and reach over your head as far as you can. Repeat five times.
7. Cervical isometrics. Press your head against your hands as follows: Do a forward press, side press, back press, and rotation press. Hold each ten seconds. Repeat each direction five times.
8. Shoulder bone. With your hands at your sides, pull your shoulder blades together in back, and tuck in your chin. Hold five seconds. Relax. Repeat five times.
9. Arm bone. Place the palms of your hands on the wall or chair in front of you. Lean toward the wall with your body, keeping hands in place. Then push back away from the wall or chair to the starting position (you may need to imagine a wall on this one). Repeat five times.
10. Goose necks. Stick your neck out (Figure 10-1), then pull it way back. The way back part is called a chin

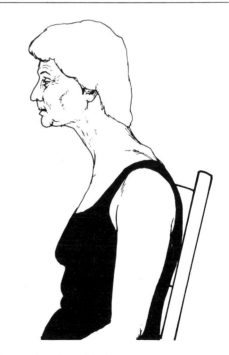

Figure 10-1 Goose Neck

tuck. This is the most important exercise you are going to learn. A chin tuck keeps your head in proper alignment. Hold the chin tuck ten seconds. Repeat ten times.

11. Shoulder shrugs. Repeat the shoulder shrugs, backward and forward, five times.

12. Face exercises. This is a fun one. We are going to make faces at each other. First, frown; then, pucker. Repeat five times.

13. Alternate arm reaches. Reach up with your right arm, and then reach up with your left arm. Then reach with your right arm, then your left arm. Repeat five times.

Remember your "do's" and "don'ts." Try to keep your neck as loose as possible by moving it often and gently. Stay in the chin tuck position as often as you can. If anything hurts, you may be progressing too fast, so slow it down.

Appendix 10-A

Nice Necks Handout

Hints

1. Support your neck at night, either with a pillow or a towel roll under your neck. Try to make your pillow provide enough support on your side so that your head is not tilted up or tilted down.
2. When working at sitting tasks, such as typing, knitting, or watching television, be aware of your neck position. Try to keep your chin tucked and your head up.
3. Try to avoid chills on your neck; wrap a towel or a scarf around your neck when in a drafty place.

Do's

1. Move your neck as often as possible.
2. Do exercises to strengthen your neck.
3. Move your head "yes" (neck flexion), "no" (rotation), "maybe" (shoulder shrug) throughout the day.

Don'ts

1. Do not move your neck in ways that are painful.
2. Do not stay in one position too long.
3. Do not sleep without supporting your neck.
4. Do not do activities that hurt your neck.
5. Do not carry heavy things when you are having neck pain, as doing so puts extra stress on your neck.

Exercises

1. Deep breaths: Repeat three times.
2. Shoulder shrugs: Repeat five times.
3. Head bends: Repeat five times.
4. Head turns: Repeat five times.
5. Head tilts: Repeat five times.
6. Arm clasp reaches: Repeat five times.
7. Cervical isometrics: Repeat each direction five times.
8. Shoulder bone: Repeat five times.
9. Arm bone: Repeat five times.
10. Goose necks: Repeat ten times.
11. Shoulder shrugs: Repeat five times.
12. Face exercises: Repeat five times.
13. Alternate arm reaches: Repeat five times.

Supple Shoulders

You are invited to attend a class on supple shoulders.

Learn about one of the most vulnerable joints in the body. Learn about bursitis, tendinitis, and rotator cuff tears. Then, learn about the correct way to exercise to keep your shoulders supple. . . .

SUPPLE SHOULDERS

at:

_____

on:

_____

in:

_____

Taught by: _____

LISTEN, LEARN, AND EXERCISE!

SUPPLE SHOULDERS

Supple Shoulders

LECTURE/DISCUSSION

The shoulder joint can be extremely troublesome because it is a very fragile and vulnerable joint. You may have heard about people who have shoulder fractures, bursitis, or tears of the muscles around the shoulder joint. This joint is susceptible to injury because of its structure. A little bony overhang that comes from the shoulder blade joins with the bone in the upper arm, called the humerus; however, there is not a direct attachment. Capsules, ligaments, and muscles, not bony structures, hold the bones of the shoulder in place. This relationship is why the force of gravity can easily pull the long arm bone down and cause problems.

One shoulder joint problem is a subluxation, which occurs when the bone in your arm pulls away from the little bony overhang. A little flat plate allows the bone in your arm to slide down as you lift your arm up (*demonstrate by raising your arm*). Many times, when people are struck in the shoulder joint, they are unable to move the arm bone down that little plate.

The biggest problem in shoulders is overuse of the muscles, leading to tendinitis around the shoulder joint where the muscle begins. Bursae, little sacs that allow the muscles to slide smoothly over each other, can also become inflamed because of excessive motion; this condition is called bursitis. In addition, people can fall and tear the muscles around the shoulder joint, as in a rotator cuff tear.

The most important thing to remember about the shoulder is that it becomes tighter and tighter when you stop moving it or using it. In addition, the position of the head can affect the movement of the shoulder. If your head is in good position, there is no problem raising your shoulders and arms all the way up in the air. If your head is forward, however, you cannot lift your shoulders and arms as well in the air (*demonstrate*). Shoulder movement is also affected by problems of the neck, which can cause pain that radiates down to your shoulders because the nerves that cause shoulder motion run through your neck muscles.

Other problems that may cause difficulty in shoulder motion are osteoarthritis and rheumatoid arthritis. These are pathological problems. Treatment for those can be gentle exercises, as well as medications prescribed by your physician.

Before you leave today, I will give each of you a handout with helpful hints for your shoulders (*Appendix 11-A; read aloud and dis-*

cuss, if desired). Now we will go through a shoulder exercise program.

EXERCISES

1. Chin tucks. Pull your head back as far as you possibly can on your shoulders like in the military (Figure 11-1). Repeat three times.
2. Shoulder rolls. Roll your shoulders around backward three times in big circles. Also roll them forward three times. Repeat three times.
3. Neck motions. Move your head in all the planes of motion. The first one is forward then back up to the middle. Repeat three times. Then move your head backward and back up to the middle. Repeat three times. Move your head side to side, trying to bring your ear to your shoulder. Repeat three times on each side. Look over your shoulder, then back toward the middle. Repeat three times in each direction.
4. Arm reaches: Reach your hands as high as possible. Reach your right hand over your left and your left hand over your right, and then bring your hands straight down. Repeat three times. Now bring your hands way out to the side, reaching as far out as you can, as if you are going to touch the sides of the walls next to you, then way up, then touch them on top of your head, and then bring them back down. Repeat three times.
5. The bell ringer. Put your arms at right angles to your shoulder, and slowly start to swing your hands back and down, then back and down again. Now relax. Repeat three times.
6. Elbow backs. Put your hands behind your neck, pull your elbows back, and then touch them in front (Figure 11-2). Repeat three times.

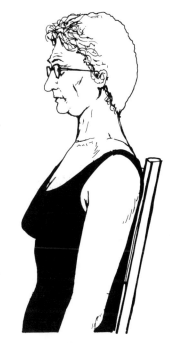

Figure 11-1 Chin Tuck

7. Forward reaches. Bring your arms forward, pointing toward the front of the room. Now stretch a little further, and relax. Repeat three times.
8. Arm back stretches. Place your hands behind your low back, and pull your hands up toward the upper part of your back as high as you can, and relax. Repeat five times.
9. Overhead ear touches. Place your forearm on your head, and try to touch your opposite ear (Figure 11-3). Then straighten your elbow. Repeat five times with each arm.
10. Hugs. Hug yourself as tight as you can around your shoulders (Figure 11-4). Relax. Repeat five times.
11. Arm circles. Put your arms out to the side, and make some small circles—three forward and three backward. Repeat three times.
12. Shoulder elbow backs. Put your hands on your shoulders, and pull your elbows back as far as you can. Relax. Repeat three times.

13. Shoulder blade backs. Pull your shoulder blades together. Hold them real tight, and then relax. Repeat three times.
14. Chicken exercises. Put your thumbs in your armpits, and flap your elbows like a chicken. Repeat three times fast, and then relax.
15. Arm shakes. Let your arms relax at your sides, and then shake them out. Repeat three times.

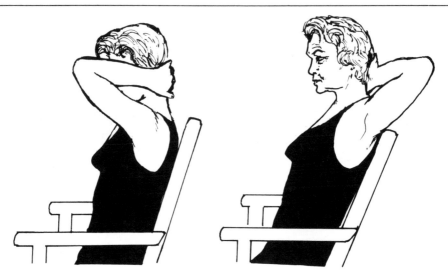

Figure 11-2 Elbow Backs

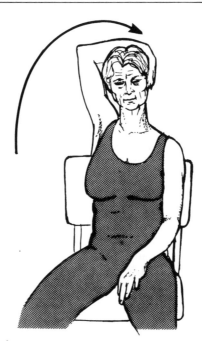

Figure 11-3 Overhead Ear Touch

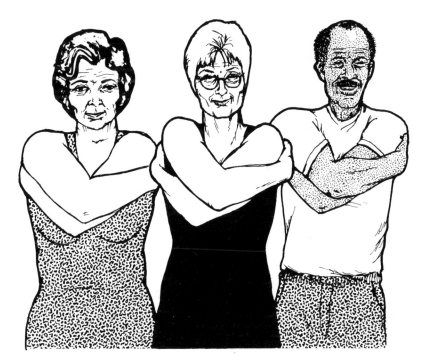

Figure 11-4 Hugs

Appendix 11-A

Supple Shoulders Handout

Hints

1. Try to keep the shoulder joints moving in pain-free ranges as much as possible.
2. Try to avoid drafts on your shoulder joints.
3. Sleep in positions that provide support to the shoulder joints.
4. Maintain good posture so that you can have good shoulder motion.

Do's

1. Swing your arms gently forward, back, and side to side three times each day to keep your shoulder joints loose.
2. Keep your shoulders warm.
3. Warm up your shoulder by exercising or applying heat before doing any strenuous activity.
4. Apply ice if you feel severe pain in your shoulder.

Don'ts

1. Do not carry objects that are too heavy.
2. Do not wear clothes that are too constricting.
3. Do not sit with your head in one position too long.
4. Do not do any activity if it hurts your shoulder joint.

Exercises

1. Chin tucks: Repeat three times.
2. Shoulder rolls: Repeat three times.
3. Neck motions: Repeat three times in each direction.
4. Arm reaches: Repeat three times.
5. The bell ringer: Repeat three times.
6. Elbow backs: Repeat three times.
7. Forward reaches: Repeat three times.
8. Arm back stretches: Repeat five times.

Agile Arms

Come learn about the exercises and the workings of your arms.

AGILE ARMS

at:

_____

on:

_____

in:

_____

Taught by: _____

LISTEN, LEARN, AND EXERCISE!

AGILE ARMS

12

Agile Arms

LECTURE/DISCUSSION

We use our arms for work and for pleasure: to carry grocery bags, pick up a grandchild, change a tire, and hug friends. What would we do without them? Not a whole lot, it seems. Has anyone here ever broken an arm? For those of you who have, I know that it was a great challenge to perform routine activities, especially if you broke your dominant arm. Ever try to brush or comb your hair with the opposite hand? You may have discovered how new hairstyles are developed!

If you discount the hand, there are actually only three bones in the arm—the humerus, the radius, and the ulna. All three bones are considered long bones. The humerus is the single bone in the upper arm. When you bang your elbow at the joint and you get that awful tingle up and down your arm, you would probably say, "I hit my funny bone." "Funny bone" is a play on words, because you have hit the ulnar nerve on the humerus bone.

At the shoulder, the head of the humerus fits into the socket of the scapula, or shoulder girdle. Of all the joints in the body, this one is at highest risk for dislocation. At the elbow, the humerus touches the two bones of the forearm, the ulna and the radius.

Mechanically, these two bones slide across each other to accommodate various movements. The top portion of the ulna can be felt in the elbow. The radius is more difficult to feel.

The muscles of the upper arm are probably some of the best known in the body. The biceps has been the indicator of strength for centuries; the triceps, on the other hand, is not so much associated with strength as with "flab." This is the muscle opposite the biceps (*indicate the areas of these muscles*). The muscles in the lower arm are less visible to the naked eye, but they have some very important tasks, such as flexing and extending the wrist and fingers, as well as moving the wrist laterally (abduction and adduction). One particular muscle flexes the hand, while another flexes the thumb.

Arm strength becomes less important for appearance and more important for function as we grow older. Barring any preexisting condition, such as moderate arthritis, multiple sclerosis, or faulty innervation to the muscles, there is no reason why we cannot maintain the integrity of the arm muscles as we grow older. Simple measures can be used to maintain and improve the integrity of these muscles. Such measures include regular isotonic exercises to improve range of motion; strength building, either through isometric exercises or through exercises with household props; and calisthenics, where medically approved.

A note of safety: if you have bursitis or any other condition that makes performing any exercise with props painful for you, do not continue the exercise. You may aggravate such a condition by doing an exercise inproperly or by doing an exercise contraindicated for your condition. Always ask your physical therapist or doctor if certain types of exercises are permissible for you.

As with other parts of your body, nonspecific pain may occasionally arise in your arm or arms. These pains may be due to fatigue, overexertion, or stress. Sometimes, it may be necessary to rest after carrying heavy packages, or a gentle massage may alleviate that dull, achy feeling. If, however, you are in an air-conditioned room or out of doors and suddenly feel your fingers lose circulation, movement of the arms is the key to the relief of that kind of pain, as the arms transport warm blood to the fingers. In this regard, the arms are very important mechanisms for people with Raynaud's disease, a disease of poor circulation.

Raising your arms above the shoulder level raises your heart rate. That is why all low- and high-impact aerobics classes emphasize arm movement as much as foot movement. Whenever you see people swinging their arms while walking, it is because this added arm movement increases the work required of the heart. Some people with heart problems should avoid raising their arms high because of this extra work that it puts on the heart.

Household props, such as soup cans of all sizes, towels, scarves, and books, can be used for arm exercises. When used safely and effectively, these props have many purposes. The cans and books, for example, provide weight. A safe amount of weight is any weight that you can lift comfortably for ten repetitions. The scarves or towels are used for flexibility exercises, mostly for the shoulder girdle. Because the shoulder is important to the arm, we will incorporate one or two shoulder exercises into this program.

I am going to give each of you a handout before you leave today so that you can review all the do's and don'ts for healthy arms and practice the exercises at home (*Appendix 12-A; read aloud and discuss if desired*). Now we are going to exercise.

EXERCISES

1. Postural check. Sit upright in your chair with your lower back supported and your weight evenly distributed on both hips.
2. Arm benders. While comfortably seated or standing, extend your arms at shoulder level. Bend your arms at the elbow to touch your shoulders, and then extend your arms. Repeat five times.
3. Small arm circles. While seated or standing, extend your arms at shoulder level. Move your arms in small circles in a clockwise direction. Do five in one direction and five in the opposite direction. Then rest your arms.
4. Biceps curls. Extend your right arm in front of you while your left arm rests on your lap. If this position is too tiring, place your exercise arm on your thigh with elbow bent. Keeping elbow stabilized, steadily curl arm up and back. A soup can may act as a weight if free weights are not available. Repeat the curl four more times (Figure 12-1); then rest for 30 seconds. Do a second set of five curls; then rest for 45 seconds. Do again; then rest. You may gradually progress to heavier weights over time, if you do this exercise three times per week. The proper weight ranges from 1 to 5 pounds for less active or nonrobust older adults.

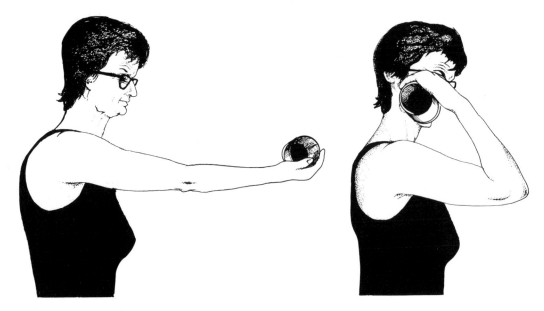

Figure 12-1 Biceps Curl

5. Front scissors. Extend your arms in front of you. Criss-cross your arms, first right arm over left, then left arm over right. Move your arms up and down (from ear position to bellybutton) at a comfortable pace. One up and down movement across the body equals one set. Repeat five times.
6. Behind scissors. Use the same criss-crossing action behind your back. Move your arms up and down while criss-crossing them.
7. Wide arm circles. Extend your arms at shoulder level. Move your arms in wide circles in a clockwise direction. Do five in this direction, and then do five in the opposite direction. Rest your arms.

Now we are going to do something different, using this army surplus parachute (or colored sheet or sail). Parachute play is demanding and may be considered an aerobic workout when used properly. The parachute may be used while you are sitting or standing. Basically, unfold the parachute, and pull it taut to provide tension. (*An adequate number of participants is necessary to achieve this.*) Once it is taut, make big and/or small waves. Walk while making waves (*if the group is standing*). We can also toss balls with the parachute or play games that involve walking under it for variety. Rolling and unrolling the parachute is excellent for lower arm and finger work, too.

Appendix 12-A

Agile Arms Handout

Do's

1. Maintain flexibility in your shoulder girdle to maintain arm movement.
2. Consider doing isolated arm exercises daily to stimulate circulation to the fingers and thumb.
3. Keep your wrist extended while using any size weight.

Don'ts

1. Do not use heavy weights when first beginning arm exercises.
2. Do not carry weights while walking without consulting your doctor if you have a heart condition or high blood pressure.
3. Do not go into damp or cold surroundings without gloves if you are prone to losing circulation in your fingers.

4. Do not pick up a glass that contains a cold drink without placing a paper napkin around the glass if you lose sensation in your fingers when touching something cold.
5. Do not grip weights too tightly; keep fingers around weight loosely.

Exercises

1. Posture check.
2. Arm benders: Repeat five times.
3. Small arm circles: Repeat five times.
4. Biceps curls: Repeat five times with each arm.
5. Front scissors: Repeat five times.
6. Behind scissors: Repeat five times.
7. Wide arm circles: Repeat five times.

Wonderful Wrists

Learn about the fascinating, yet tiny, wrist joint.

WONDERFUL WRISTS

at:

_____

on:

_____

in:

_____

Taught by: _____

LISTEN, LEARN, AND EXERCISE!

WONDERFUL WRISTS

13

Wonderful Wrists

LECTURE/DISCUSSION

We do not usually think about our wrists until they start to hurt. It is not uncommon for our wrists to hurt or bother us, however, if we overuse them. One thing that we want to do today is to make sure that you have good strong wrists and that you are using them to the best of your ability. To check them, turn to your neighbors, and shake their hands. Notice how your wrist moves when you do this.

The wrist joint is a very complex joint. It is made up of the two bones in your forearm, as well as the tiny bones at the bottom part of your hand. The wrist does not just bend forward and backward; it also turns your hand at the elbow (*demonstrate*). Try these different motions with your wrists. Bend your hand back, and then bend your hand down. Now turn your hand at the elbow. These motions are called flexion, extension, pronation, and supination. If these motions become difficult, you will have trouble with many types of daily activities, such as writing, driving a car, getting dressed, and even turning doorknobs.

Also part of the wrist joint anatomy are muscles that go across the joint. Most of the wrist joint is composed of tendons, so it is not uncommon to have tendinitis at the wrist or elbow and to have some problems with compression of blood vessels and nerves at that space. You may have heard of people who have carpal tunnel syndrome, a tightness or constriction in the tissue on the palmar part of the wrist. This causes a decrease in motion in either bending or extending, which can result in significant pain down into the fingers. Besides surgery, the best treatment for carpal tunnel syndrome is to avoid excessive motions. Riding a bicycle, which entails leaning on your hands, can cause significant pain for people who have carpal tunnel syndrome. Arthritis can also involve the wrist. Again, monitored safe exercise programs help tremendously with this. It is very important to take care of your wrists and slowly strengthen them.

Before you leave today, I am going to give each of you a list of do's and don'ts, with some helpful hints, for healthy wrists (*Appendix 13-A; read aloud and discuss, if desired*).

EXERCISES

1. Wrist bends. Rest your forearms on the chair arms, and bend your wrist down so that your fingers point to the floor. Take a look at your wrists and compare the two together. See how

74

far they go. Now turn your palms to the ceiling, and see if you can point your fingers straight up. Repeat ten times.

2. Wrist pushes. Gently grasp your right hand and push your left wrist down. Push so that your palm is coming down to the ground. Hold ten seconds. Then push your right wrist down with your left hand. Repeat three times.

3. Palm turns. Put your elbows in at your side. Turn one hand palm up, then palm down. Repeat three times.

4. Wrist wiggles. Clasp your hands together, and wiggle your wrists. Make like you are a fish in the sea going through the water. Wiggle your hands forward away from your body, and wiggle them back toward your body. Repeat ten times.

5. Wrist circles. With each wrist, make big round circles. Repeat ten times with each wrist.

6. Thumb lifts. Let your arms rest on the arms of the chair, and raise your thumbs toward the ceiling. Now lift your thumbs all the way up toward the ceiling. Do this on both hands. Repeat ten times.

7. Baby finger lifts. Turn your hand so that your thumb side is down. Lift the baby finger of your hand toward the ceiling. Repeat three times with each hand.

8. Wrist lifts and falls. Rest your arm flat so that your palm is facing the ground and let your hand hang over the chair arm. Lift the back of your hand up toward the ceiling, and let it fall back down. Repeat three times with each hand.

As you see, the wrist program does not take that long. You can go through the entire exercise program in about ten minutes.

Appendix 13-A

Wonderful Wrists Handout

Hints

1. Avoid carrying heavy objects.
2. Alternate activities. For example, if you always open a door with your right hand, try opening it with your left hand so that you are using a different motion. You can also do this with jars.
3. Avoid leaning on your wrists, as this may cause excessive pressure.

Do's

1. Exercise your wrists regularly.
2. Stretch your wrists as often as possible.
3. Heat your wrists up before doing activities.
4. Put ice on your wrists if they hurt after exercise.

Don'ts

1. Do not carry heavy items with your wrists either in severe flexion or in severe extension.
2. Do not sleep with your wrists in severe flexion or severe extension.

Exercises

1. Wrist bends: Repeat ten times.
2. Wrist pushes: Do three times.
3. Palm turns: Do three times.
4. Wrist wiggles: Repeat ten times.
5. Wrist circles: Repeat ten times with each wrist.
6. Thumb lifts: Repeat ten times.
7. Baby finger lifts: Repeat three times.
8. Wrist lifts and falls: Repeat three times with each wrist.

14

Hardy Hands and Flexible Fingers

Look at your hands and fingers. What do you see?

Come and learn the answer at a class on . . .

HARDY HANDS AND FLEXIBLE FINGERS

at:

_____

on:

_____

in:

_____

Taught by: _____

LISTEN, LEARN, AND EXERCISE!

HARDY HANDS AND FLEXIBLE FINGERS

14

Hardy Hands and Flexible Fingers

LECTURE/DISCUSSION

When you look at your hands and fingers, you can see tendons. Those are the rubbery, hard-looking things running into each finger. You can see blood vessels, probably veins, and you can see muscles, mostly on the palmar side of your hand, where there is much more muscle bulk.

Look at the movement of your fingers and hand. If you make a tight fist, you can see that your fingers flex. Then straighten your fingers out, and you can see that your fingers extend. If they are healthy, they actually go a few degrees past a neutral position at the palm joint, called the metacarpal joint (*show the joint*). Now take a look at your thumb. Bring it around in a big circle (*demonstrate*). You can see that the thumb goes around in a big circle and bends down. You can touch your baby finger. In fact, the thumb is the only finger that can touch all your other fingers by itself (*demonstrate*). Your hands also do something very interesting. Put your fingers together, and spread your fingers apart. This motion is called finger abduction, and it is what accentuates some of that muscle bulk in the palm of your hand.

The fingers have several long bones that run from approximately the middle of your palm to the end of your fingers. You can see

where each finger bone ends and makes separate joints with other bones in each finger. Part of the reason that the hands can be so painful when people have a disease in them is the fact that there are so many joints in the hands. Each of those joints is a tiny capsule that, like the larger joints, has a cover, or capsule, tendons, and muscles. There are a few muscles in the finger joints, but most of the hand is made up of tendons that come from the lower arm. There are also ligaments that hold the joints together at each bend in the finger.

One of the problems that occur in the hand is arthritis. There are two types of arthritis: osteoarthritis and rheumatoid arthritis. Osteoarthritis, which affects one or two joints, is usually a wear-and-tear type problem that happens in the hands. People who have been typists or piano players are usually more prone to osteoarthritis, for example. The pain is in the distal joints, that is, the joints farther away from the arm. The best thing that you can do for osteoarthritis is rest and not work the joints too hard.

Rheumatoid arthritis is a whole body disease. It affects more than just the hand. When it gets into the hands, it is in the joint closest to your palm. The hands may become red, swollen, and inflamed. For this type of arthritis, you also need to rest, but, when the hand begins to feel better, you really need to begin to work it and use the muscles in your hand.

You can also get tendinitis in the hand. Sometimes, as people get older, they get contractures and scarring in the palms and surface of their hands, although no one is sure why. Some people have a temporary problem with their hands called synovitis. The joints become a little swollen and tender from overuse, such as writing too much. The best treatment for synovitis is to rest and to use heat or ice to relieve some of the inflammation.

I will give you a handout with some helpful hints and some do's and don'ts for healthy hands before you leave today (*Appendix 14-A; read aloud and discuss, if desired*). Now, we are going to exercise our hands and fingers.

EXERCISES

1. Finger touches. First, touch your thumb to each of the fingers in your hand. Start from the index finger, and go down to the ring finger. Now go back the other way—baby finger, ring finger, middle finger, index finger, thumb. Repeat five times in each direction with each hand.
2. Thumb circles. Make a big circle with each thumb. Repeat five times.
3. Thumb tips. Bend the tip of your thumb, and straighten it out. Repeat five times with each thumb.
4. Finger spreads. Spread your fingers apart, and then bring them back together (Figure 14-1). Repeat ten times.
5. Palm joint bends. Bend your fingers at the joint closest to the palm, keeping all the other joints straight. Repeat ten times.
6. Finger tip bends. Bend the tips of your fingers, keeping the other joints straight, and then straighten the tips. Repeat three times.
7. Fists. Make a tight fist, and then open your hand. Repeat three times with each hand.

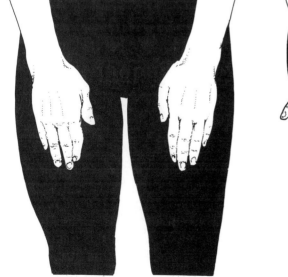
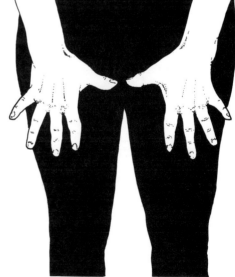

Figure 14-1 Finger Spreads

8. Palm presses. Put your two hands together, and press them gently together. Repeat three times.
9. Backhand presses. Put the backs of your hands together, starting with your fingertips and going all the way up to your wrists. Then gently push off the backs of your hands. Repeat three times.
10. Finger presses. Put your two hands together, and push the two hands against each other at the baby finger; do the same at the ring finger. Repeat three times.
11. Itsy Bitsy Spider. Touch your left index finger to your right thumb and your left thumb to your right index finger. Then rotate around the thumb to the index finger and the index finger to the thumb so that the spider is climbing upward (Figure 14-2). Repeat ten times.
12. Play the piano. Roll your fingers like you are playing the piano, back and forth. Repeat five times.
13. Waves. Pretend your hands are waves moving up and down like a wave wiggling your fingers. Repeat ten times.
14. Hand shakes. Shake your hands out. Repeat five times.

Now we are going to repeat the exercises, starting from the end and going back up to the beginning. Be sure to shake out your hands after every three exercises while doing them with music.

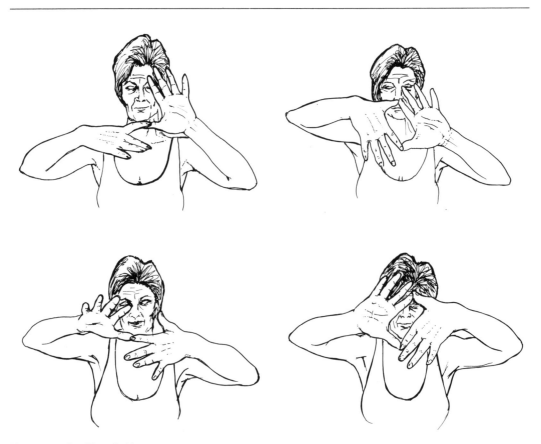

Figure 14-2 Itsy Bitsy Spider

Appendix 14-A

Hardy Hands and Flexible Fingers Handout

Hints

1. Every once in a while, stretch your hands and fingers.
2. Avoid excessive pressure or stress on your hands.
3. If you find that your hands feel better when they are warm, wear gloves.
4. Try to avoid awkward positions for your hand.

Do's

1. Exercise your hand as much as possible.
2. Spread your fingers apart and together as often as possible.
3. If your hands hurt, decrease the number of activities that require you to use them.
4. If your hand activities are excessive, apply ice afterward.
5. Warm your hands by placing them in warm water if you are going to use them a great deal.
6. Shake out your hands if you have been using them excessively.
7. Massage your hands if they hurt.

Don'ts

1. Do not carry heavy items.

2. Do not hold your hand in one position for too long.
3. Do not let people shake your hand too hard if your hand hurts.
4. Do not use ice or heat if it irritates your hands and makes them feel worse.

Exercises

1. Finger touches: Repeat five times in each direction.
2. Thumb circles: Repeat five times.
3. Thumb tips: Repeat five times.
4. Finger spreads: Repeat ten times.
5. Palm joint bends: Repeat ten times.
6. Finger tip bends: Repeat three times.
7. Fists: Repeat three times.
8. Palm presses: Repeat three times.
9. Backhand presses: Repeat three times.
10. Finger presses: Repeat three times.
11. Itsy Bitsy Spider: Repeat ten times.
12. Play the piano: Repeat five times.
13. Waves: Repeat ten times.
14. Hand shakes: Repeat five times.

15

Improving Balance

Do you have a problem with balance?

Did you know that falls due to balance are one of the major reasons older persons are admitted to hospitals?

Don't become a hospital statistic.

Come to the class on . . .

IMPROVING BALANCE

at:

_____

on:

_____

in:

_____

Taught by: _____

LISTEN, LEARN, AND EXERCISE!

IMPROVING BALANCE

15

Improving Balance

LECTURE/DISCUSSION

No one wants to go into a hospital. Falls are one of the main reasons that older persons are admitted to the hospital or nursing homes.

Geriatric researchers agree that about one-third of people over the age of 65 have one or more falls in a year resulting in almost 10,000 deaths. Injuries from falls are the sixth leading cause of death in people over the age of 75.

These accidents, many of which are preventable, take a devastating toll on older persons. These older people may suffer life-threatening complications while other older people develop limitation of activity, dependence, and unhappiness. Many older people are prevented from living at home because of potentially treatable imbalance problems.

My many years of clinical experience with older persons have borne out time and time again that if older persons took care of their bodies by stretching and strengthening muscles, a physical therapist would not see so many older persons with fractured hips and balance problems.

Source: Reprinted from *Self Balance Hints for Older Persons*, Carole B. Lewis, an Aspen Consumer Information Pamphlet, © 1987 by Aspen Publishers, Inc.

Developing flexibility is one way of keeping fit and avoiding balance problems. Developing strength in muscle groups is a second line of defense.

In this class, we will do stretching and strengthening exercises that I consider to be extremely important in an older person's body to make it strong, flexible, and more coordinated. In addition, I will discuss ways of improving posture. Before we begin the exercises, I would like us to do a short self-test.

There are several ingredients that make a person more at risk for falls and balance problems. Some of the major ingredients are posture, blood regulations, brain input, strength, flexibility, and the environment.

To check if posture is a problem, we must first be aware of good posture.

In good posture, an imaginary line goes through your ear, shoulder, hip, and knee. (*Show them.*) In abnormal or potentially problematic posture, a person's head or trunk may be in front of this line (*show them and tell participants to look at their handout [Appendix 15-A]*).

(*Have the participants stand and either you or they can quickly look for posture problems. Remember to give lots of positive reinforcement for good aspects of posture. Tell them you will be doing exercises today to improve and maintain posture.*)

Blood Flow

Sometimes the heart is unable to get blood to the brain as quickly as it is needed. To check if this is a problem, tonight, with a friend watching, lie down and sit up quickly. If you feel light-headed or dizzy, this is a sign that you may have some difficulty in this area. If the problem is severe, consult your physician. If it is only mild, make a commitment to yourself to sit or stand still for one to two minutes every time you change position before getting up or walking to allow your blood to get to the brain.

Nerve Input

If we stop moving our necks because of jobs or habit, the brain will get less information on our neck and body position. If you notice that you turn your whole body instead of your head when you look around, you may need more stimulation to the nerve endings in your neck. One way to get this is, before getting out of bed in the morning and before falling asleep at night, gently rock your head back and forth for one to two minutes. This should be done every day and you will not see the effects for several months.

Strength

Weakness in your legs can be a very important factor in loss of balance. If you are very weak in your hips or thighs, you should see a physical therapist to design an exercise program to improve your muscle strength. The foot and lower leg strength is often the key culprit and can be easily assessed and treated. Try to hop on one foot; if you cannot do this, this may be muscle weakness. To strengthen these muscles, simply go up and down on your toes. Start with 10; progress by increments of 10 a week until you reach 100. We will do this exercise today.

Flexibility

Flexibility as with strength is very important for good balance. If you are very tight, consult a physical therapist. Again, legs and feet are often overlooked and are very important. To check this area, stand leaning forward toward your chair, keeping your heels flat. If your back heel does not touch the floor, this indicates tightness. We will do exercises later for this. Another tight area is the hips. Stand in front of a mirror, and try to make a circle with your hips without moving your shoulders. As you do this, look in the mirror. If your shoulders move, you need to work on this. The exercise for this is to slowly practice these circles in front of the mirror without moving your shoulders. We will do this exercise later, too.

One last thing before we begin the exercises. If you have any existing medical problems or if any of the exercises that we do produce pain, *do not continue* with them. Consult your physical therapist or physician. First, I will show you the exercise. Then we will do it together. After we have done all the exercises this way, we will run through the exercises twice to music. We will begin the exercises now.

EXERCISES

1. Deep breaths. Take three big relaxing breaths.
2. Chin tucks. Stand as erect as you can, and gently tuck in your chin so that you create a straight line from your ear to your shoulders. Repeat three times, relaxing, breathing, and holding for ten seconds. Be sure to hold the position, not your breath.
3. Shoulder backs. Pull your shoulders back as if you had a piece of elastic pulling your shoulder blades together in the back. Hold that for ten seconds, and relax. Repeat three times, relaxing, breathing, and holding the position for ten seconds.

4. Shoulder shrugs. Bring your shoulders around in big circles, three times forwards and three times backwards.
5. Head rocks. Gently rock your head from side to side ten times. It is good to do this exercise before you get out of bed in the morning and before you go to sleep at night.
6. Back flatteners. Flatten your lower back against the chair. Hold ten seconds, and relax. Repeat five times.
7. Seated hip circles. Make a circle with your hips five times in each direction.
8. Knee strengtheners. Extend your leg from the knee. Hold for five seconds. Repeat five times.
9. Knee rolls. With your legs straight, roll your knees out and in ten times (Figure 15-1).
10. Knee bends. Bend your knees as high as you can five times each.
11. Ankle bends. Bend your ankles up and down ten times.
12. Ankle circles. Make big circles with your ankles ten times in each direction.
13. Toe curls and straighteners. Curl and straighten your toes ten times.
14. Toe ups. Go up on your toes as high as you can; come back down. Do this ten times, increasing each week five times until you build up to fifty.
15. Heel cord stretch. With your hands on the chair, keeping your heels flat, lean into the wall so that you feel a stretch in your calf muscles; hold for 30 seconds.
16. Leg lifts. Stand up, and gently swing your leg back and forth ten times. Then out to the side and back. Repeat ten times.
17. Side leg lifts. Gently swing your leg out to the side and back ten times.
18. Hip clocks. Stand in front of your mirror, and make a big circle with your hips as if there is a clock around your feet, going around to one, two, three, four, etc. until you have made a clockwise direction; then go counterclockwise, trying not to move your shoulders. Repeat five times.
19. Gluteal sets. Pinch your buttocks together. Hold five seconds. Then relax; repeat ten times.
20. Deep breaths. While standing, take three deep relaxing breaths.

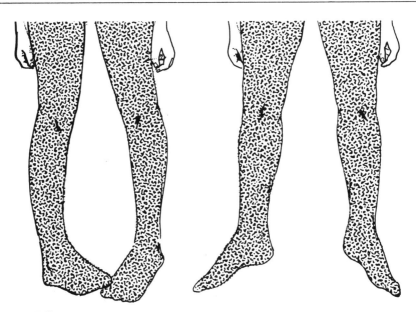

Figure 15-1 Knee Rolls

Appendix 15-A

Improving Balance Handout

Do's

1. Stretch and move as often as possible. When watching television, stand up, and move your hips during commercials (this will keep you more flexible).
2. Make sure your house is well lit (poor lighting can cause you not to see a potential hazard).
3. Focus on a far object when you walk (this will help your visual balance).
4. Lean into forces. For example, if the wind is blowing, lean into it (this will give you balance advantage).
5. Do the exercises daily, and be patient (you may not see results for three months).

Don'ts

1. Do not get up too quickly; getting up quickly can cause dizziness.
2. Do not go out into bright sunlight from a dark area without sunglasses (glare can affect your balance).
3. Do not push yourself if you feel tired (pushing yourself when you are tired can overexert your system and cause you to fall).

Exercises

1. Deep breaths: Take three big relaxing breaths.
2. Chin tucks: Repeat three times.
3. Shoulder backs: Repeat three times.
4. Shoulder shrugs: Repeat three times forwards and backwards.
5. Head rocks: Repeat ten times.
6. Back flatteners: Repeat five times.
7. Seated hip circles: Do five times in each direction.
8. Knee strengtheners: Repeat five times.
9. Knee rolls: Repeat ten times.
10. Knee bends: Do five times with each leg.

11. Ankle bends: Do ten times with each ankle.
12. Ankle circles: Do ten times in each direction.
13. Toe curls and straighteners: Repeat ten times.
14. Toe ups: Do this ten times, increasing each week five times until you build up to fifty.
15. Heel cord stretch: Hold for thirty seconds.
16. Leg lifts: Repeat ten times.
17. Side leg lifts: Repeat ten times.
18. Hip clocks: Repeat five times.
19. Gluteal sets: Repeat ten times.
20. Deep breaths: While standing, take three deep relaxing breaths.

Realizing Relaxation

Relaxation is a luxury, but it is something that can be more beneficial to you than some of the most expensive luxuries around.

Come and learn how to relax in a fun-filled class on . . .

REALIZING RELAXATION

at:

_____

on:

_____

in:

_____

Taught by: _____

LISTEN, LEARN, AND EXERCISE!

REALIZING RELAXATION

16

Realizing Relaxation

LECTURE/DISCUSSION

Relaxing is not as easy as it sounds. Many people who have lived each day wound tighter than a spring think of relaxing their minds and bodies as a difficult task. Relaxation is an art. We often think of relaxation as sleep, a vacation, or a solitary walk in the garden or around the block. In some cultures, it is part of an accepted daily routine; in our highly pressured and bottom-line society, it is a luxury.

Recognizing the need to relax is important, but before we talk about relaxation, consider the feeling of stress. Many of you have said that you recognize negative stressors, which bring on negative emotions, such as anger, sadness, or depression. Positive stressors can also produce feelings of anxiety and stress, however. For example, every bride feels happy and excited, but this very happiness and excitement can cause weight loss or weight gain, disturbances in sleep patterns, skin irritations, and the like. These are some of the ways that our bodies let us know that we need to take care of ourselves before stress causes more profound problems.

The warning signs of stress include physical symptoms, emotional reactions, and certain actions or behaviors. The easiest to detect are physical symptoms, such as tightness in the neck and shoulders; high blood pressure; fatigue; a burning sensation in the pit of the stomach; irritated bowels; and grinding teeth, especially while asleep. Emotional reactions range from anger, depression, and irritability to total apathy. These emotions are manifested through behavior, such as under- or overeating; disturbed sleep patterns (i.e., sleeping more may be a sign of depression); absent-mindedness; increased reliance on drugs, including alcohol, to feel "good"; or occasional outbursts of tears because of a sudden feeling of being overwhelmed. So, recognizing the symptoms of stress is the first step toward relaxation.

Relaxation is important basically because it has a positive effect on the body. Blood pressure has been known to drop, increased heart rates can be lowered, headaches can be alleviated or sometimes made to go away, and the production of endorphins can be increased. Some of these results can be obtained without medication, if the proper technique is used consistently over an extended period of time. Such behaviors as having a drink (whether it be coffee, tea, or alcohol), watching television, or eating do not reverse the negative effects of stressors in our daily lives. Relaxation is a skill that must be learned.

True relaxation has several goals. One is to release tension and stress in various parts of the body. Another is to reduce irritability, nervousness, and anxiety. Some of the relaxation techniques that older adults have found to be useful include progressive muscular relaxation, visual imagery, and pet therapy. Depending on the type of relaxation exercise, concentration skills may be improved. This is most likely to happen with the use of visual imagery or meditation.

Progressive muscular relaxation is a technique that many people use, often without knowing that they are using it.* Anytime you squeeze a certain body part and then release the tension, you are performing the first stage of this technique. The important points to remember are (1) take a relaxed position, but not one where you will fall asleep; (2) never hold your breath during these exercises; and (3) concentrate on the feeling of releasing the tension from various parts of your body, *not* on squeezing too tightly.

EXERCISES

Progressive Muscular Relaxation

Sit up comfortably, and close your eyes. Take a nice deep breath, and relax. Again, take a nice deep breath while calmly sitting comfortably in your chair. We are going to start with the muscles at the top of your head and end with those at the tips of your toes. Remember to breathe normally throughout this exercise.

---

*Caution: This technique has been known to raise blood pressure to dangerous levels or cause undue stress to the body because of the decreased capacity of some older adults to recover adequately from vasoconstriction.

Pretend that it is a warm sunny day and that the sun is in your eyes. Squint your eyes, squeezing the lids tightly. Let all the tension in your forehead, mouth, and jaws be channeled into the squint. Hold the tension. Feel the discomfort. Now relax the tightness around your eyes. Release all the tension from your face, forehead, and jaw. Continue to breathe comfortably and deeply.

Now, let us work on the tension in your neck and shoulders. Pull your shoulders way up, squeezing the shoulder blades together as you feel the tension building. Hold that position for five seconds as you squeeze at about 70 percent of your maximum force. One, two, three, four, five. Begin to relax, slowly lowering your shoulders and relaxing your shoulder blades. Release all of the tension from your neck and shoulders, and continue to breathe deeply and slowly.

With both hands resting in your lap, make fists. Squeeze gently while you think of all the annoying things in your life. As you think, feel the tension in your upper arms, your forearms, your wrists, thumbs, and fingers begin to build. The fists that you made contain much of the impatience and annoyances in your daily life. Feel that tension; now slowly start to release it. Let your fingers unfold; let your thumbs, forearms, and upper arms relax. Enjoy the sensation of relaxation, calmness, and peacefulness that the lack of tension brings. Continue to breathe deeply and calmly.

Moving down the body, as you continue to breathe deeply and calmly, begin to contract the muscles in your stomach. Do not squeeze to the point of discomfort, but squeeze just enough to mimic the tightness that you sometimes feel when under stress. Concentrate on your stomach muscles. Now, add your buttocks muscles. Squeeze them together, slowly building the tension in the lower area of your body. Your stomach and buttocks muscles should feel tense and firm as you concentrate. Continue to breathe calmly. Now, slowly relax your buttocks muscles. Feel the comfort of the nice soft cushion on which you are sitting. Now, relax your stomach muscles. Enjoy the calmness and lack of tension. As you breathe deeply and slowly, think of calmness and relaxation.

As you sit there, feel the constraints of your shoes on your toes. Curl your toes under, flexing the muscles in the bottoms of your feet. Feel the tension and fatigue in your feet that come from walking all day or from shoes that are too tight, corns that hurt, or bunions that ache. Let all the tension your feet produce curl up your toes. Hold that feeling. Let go of all the tension in your feet, especially your toes. Breathe calmly, quietly, and deeply. Feel how relaxed the body can become after hard work and much tension. Relish the calmness, and enjoy the quietude (*silence for a minute*). Now, begin to open your eyes.

Imagery

The next exercise that we are going to do is called guided or visual imagery. Visual or mental imagery became quite popular with professional athletes and with those in the medical community. (It was discovered that visualizing good cells fighting bad cells can help to keep disease, even cancer, in check or improve a patient's chance of recovery.) Imagery has also been found to be effective as a stress management tool in reducing blood pressure.

I will guide you through an imaginary trip that you will create. Only you will know if you are effectively visualizing the scenes as I describe them. If you have trouble concentrating, just sit back, breathe deeply, and concentrate on my voice.

I will guide you into an image that will be relaxing and warm. It is important that you associate that image with deep relaxation. It is also important that you see yourself in that image. Before I begin, is there anyone here who absolutely hates the beach or is afraid of the ocean? I want to know what

kind of an image to describe. You will have to help me (*entertain other ideas if anyone in the class objects to the ocean scenario*).

Begin by once again closing your eyes while sitting comfortably. Take a deep breath, and slowly let it out. You are beginning to feel warm and calm. Take another deep breath, and this time, as you inhale, smell the salt of the ocean. The smell brings to you images of warm sunshine, soft sand beneath your feet, and the cries of sea gulls circling above. Breathe that fresh, salty air, and feel the sunshine (*pause*). Imagine yourself in a quiet spot, sitting under a beach umbrella, watching the waves lap upon the shore. Hear the roar of the ocean; feel the coolness of the spray. You feel warm, calm, and peaceful in this quiet spot. The sky is clear and blue with scattered wisps of clouds. An occasional passing ship can be seen in the not-too-distant horizon (*pause*). You are warm, calm, and peaceful. You feel serene, happy, and at peace. The warm breeze envelopes your body, and the sun shines generously upon your chair. As you see yourself sitting, you think about the sea gulls bobbing up and down and wonder what it would be like to float aimlessly and carefree in the blue-green, transparent waters. You see yourself floating. Your body is buoyant, light, and supported by the tepid, blue-green waters. Experience the feeling of lightness, where all tension is released from your body. See yourself basking in the sunlight, dreamily floating in safe, warm waters (*pause*). As you float on, the sun's brightness begins to dim. You return to your beach chair and wrap yourself in a warm, fluffy terrycloth bathrobe to dry. You sit upright, aware of dusk approaching. As the sun begins to set and the warm breeze turns a little cooler, you briskly walk along the shore. It begins to darken, and the moon rises. You are alert and refreshed. You are calm and peaceful in this quietude. Whenever you are ready, please open your eyes (*ask whether the class enjoyed the exercise, and discuss the fact that not all techniques are for everyone*).

Pet Therapy

The final relaxation technique that I would like to share with you is a passive one. Many times we take things for granted. Little did we know 20 years ago that pets would be as healthy for us as we now know them to be. For example, studies have shown that owning a pet can reduce milder levels of stress. In fact, blood pressure is known to decrease in those who sit for regular, short intervals and watch fish swim in their tanks. Owners of dogs, cats, and birds have been observed to have lower anxiety levels, fewer bouts of loneliness, and lower blood pressures. So, if relaxation is something you must build toward, you might want to consider owning a goldfish or two, just to watch, talk to, or take care of. I will give you a handout today with some helpful hints and reminders of what we have discussed about relaxation (*Appendix 16-A; review if desired*).

Appendix 16-A

Realizing Relaxation Handout

Hints

1. Relaxation is a learned behavior. Give your body time to learn to relax, do not rush any one technique.
2. Choose a relaxation technique that will work for you. Not everyone can practice the same technique. Although imagery may work for some, a more physical exercise, such as tai chi or progressive muscular relaxation, may be best for others.
3. Learn to breathe deeply and slowly. Shallow breathing is a sign of anxiety or an aroused state. Also, shallow breathing does not supply the most effective amount of oxygen to surrounding tissue.
4. Practice relaxation at the same time every day. Consistency builds habit, and continuous skill development is the key to good results.

Do's

1. Consider giving yourself an occasional foot massage, taking a warm bath, and listening to symphonic music as additions to your stress reduction repertoire.
2. Purchase relaxation audiotapes on which a speaker conducts visual imagery. Some tapes may have subliminal messages to boost self-image and positive thoughts, but there is no harm in these materials.
3. Experiment with different modes of relaxation. Yoga, tai chi, rolfing, and massage have all been used successfully by a variety of individuals. The instructor should be certified in all cases. Do not hesitate to inquire about the training of any person who is conducting relaxation techniques.
4. Practice regularly and consistently.
5. Practice positive thinking. For example, say to yourself "calm down" or "I am strong, I am calm" or "I am warm and safe."
6. Keep everyday events in perspective. Avoid placing unnecessary stress on yourself by overreacting to a situation.
7. Always try to find humor in life's daily happenings. Humor is a panacea to everyday frustrations.

8. Try to keep a positive attitude. No one enjoys a negative person.

Don'ts

1. Do not use moderate or strenuous exercise as a relaxation technique. Remember, you are trying to relax the muscles, not contract them.
2. Do not use alcohol, nicotine, or other drugs to relax you. Learn to relax yourself. Give your body the right to control its reactions.
3. Do not take part in any activity in which you do not feel comfort-able. If you do not like yoga after the first few sessions in which you participate, do not continue. However, distinguish between not giving something a chance and truly disliking it.
4. Do not buy a young pet with the immediate hope that it will help you relax. Remember that kittens and puppies need to be toilet-trained. House-trained pets may be best for you if you are impatient and dislike surprises.
5. Do not expect other people to relax you. Only you can effect that response in your body.

Abatable Arthritis

Did you know that 50 percent of the people over 65 years of age and 75 percent of the people over 80 years of age have arthritis?

Did you also know that *proper* exercise can help?

Come learn what can be done for . . .

ABATABLE ARTHRITIS

at:

_____

on:

_____

in:

_____

Taught by: _____

LISTEN, LEARN, AND EXERCISE!

ABATABLE ARTHRITIS

Abatable Arthritis

LECTURE/DISCUSSION

The sad fact is that 50 percent of the people over 65 years of age and 75 percent of the people over 80 years of age have osteoarthritis. Many rheumatologists believe that everybody who lives long enough will eventually have arthritis. However, it is possible to cope with arthritis if you can work systematically on a good exercise program. The word *arthritis* comes from *arth*, meaning joint, and *ritis*, meaning inflammation. A joint is the place where two bones meet. Each joint has cartilage to help the bones move across each other smoothly. Muscles go around the bones as nice even levers so that people can move freely through their activities.

There are two major kinds of arthritis: osteoarthritis and rheumatoid arthritis. Osteoarthritis affects one or two joints, usually a knee, a shoulder, or a hip. Some studies have shown that the more stress put on a joint, the worse the arthritis becomes. For example, many people believe that runners are prone to arthritis in the knee, while piano players and typists may have arthritis in the fingers. To date, however, this has not been definitively

proved. Even so, it seems wise to avoid excessive stress on any joints. Because the major shock-absorbing mechanism of the joint is not, in fact, the cartilage, which is destroyed in osteoarthritis, but muscle, and because muscle can absorb up to 80 percent of the shock, strengthening the muscles around the joint affected by osteoarthritis can take away some of the shock. Strengthening the muscles in the knee, for example, will make it easier for a person to bear weight on that knee when walking. That is the aim of many of the exercises that we will be doing today.

Rheumatoid arthritis is a systemic disease that affects multiple joints. With rheumatoid arthritis, the capsule around the joint becomes inflamed and swollen. The person may have pain and swelling in many joints (e.g., in the hip, the knee, the shoulder, and the hands), as well as fatigue. This kind of arthritis is associated with deformities of the hands much more than is osteoarthritis. People who have rheumatoid arthritis can also benefit from exercise, but they must exercise when they have the least amount of pain in their joints. They make dramatic improvements, however. Muscles can help to move the joint more freely if they are stretched and strong, which is why we are going to do exercises. For more detailed information, you may want to contact the Arthritis Foundation; most cities have a local chapter.

Before we do these exercises, I am going to give you a handout with some general hints for dealing with arthritis (*Appendix 17-A; read aloud and discuss, if desired*).

EXERCISES

1. Deep breaths. Take three deep breaths three times.
2. Chin tucks. Tuck in your chin and lift up the back of your head three times.
3. Head motions. Do three times each.
   (a) side to side
   (b) over each shoulder.
4. Shoulder circles. Make three circles backward with your shoulders and three circles forward with your shoulders.
5. Shoulder shrugs. Do three times.
6. Arm reaches. With your arms out in front reach as far forward as you can, repeat this exercise to the side, backward, and down to the floor. Do this three times in each direction.
7. Shake out. With your arms hanging at your sides, shake out your arms so that they relax. Do this for ten seconds.
8. Hands behind head. Do this exercise three times. Place your hands behind your head and pull your elbows apart, bring your elbows back in.

9. The elbow exerciser.
   (a) bend your elbow up and down three times
   (b) turn your palm up and down three times
10. Wrist exerciser. Bend your wrist up and down three times.
11. Hand exerciser. Make a tight fist with your hand and then stretch your fingers way out.
12. Finger wiggler. Wiggle your fingers for ten seconds.
13. Finger toucher. Touch the tip of your thumb to each of your fingers, go all the way down and come all the way back. Do this three times.
14. Point exercise. Sitting in the chair, put your hands in the small of your back and gently arch your back, then gently tilt your trunk to each side and gently turn your trunk over each shoulder. Do each of these three times.
15. Hip rocks. Gently lift up on your hips in the chair with one hip and then the other. Do this three times with each hip.
16. Leg exercisers. Straighten your legs out and twist your knee out with your leg straight. Do this three times.
17. Leg shake out. Shake your legs out, get them all relaxed all the way up to your hips.
18. Ankle bends. Three times each. Ankle circle three times each.
19. Toe bends. Curl your toes as tight as you can.
20. Toe spreads. Spread your toes as far apart as you can. Three times each.

Appendix 17-A

Abatable Arthritis Handout

Hints

1. Try to do short bouts of exercise as often as possible.
2. If you hurt in a joint for more than an hour after an activity, you may have done too much. Next time, do only half as much, and increase the exertion slowly each time.
3. Sit, stand, and sleep in comfortable, supported positions. If you get up from a position sore, it was not good for you.

Do's

1. Warm up your joints before exercising, either with a heating pad or with five minutes of slow, gentle movement.
2. Swim as often as possible.

Don'ts

1. Do not stay in one position too long.
2. Do not wear tight elastic wraps around painful joints.
3. Do not vibrate an arthritic joint.

Exercises

1. Deep breaths. Three times.
2. Chin tucks. Three times.
3. Head motions. Three times each.
4. Shoulder circles. Three circles backward and forward.
5. Shoulder shrugs. Three times.
6. Arm reaches. Three times each in each direction.
7. Shake out. Do for ten seconds.
8. Hands behind head. Three times.
9. The elbow exerciser. Elbow up three times. Palm up three times.
10. Wrist exerciser. Up and down three times.
11. Hand exerciser. Make a tight fist with your hands and then stretch your fingers way out.
12. Finger wiggler. Wiggle your finger for ten seconds.
13. Finger toucher. Do three times.
14. Pointer exerciser. Do three times.
15. Hip rocks. Do three times.
16. Leg exerciser. Do three times.
17. Leg shake out. Shake your legs out, get them all relaxed all the way up to your hips.
18. Ankle bends. Do three times.
19. Toe bends. Curl your toes as tight as you can.
20. Toe spreads. Do three times.

Preventing Parkinson's Problems

Parkinson's disease can be very debilitating. However, a home exercise program can keep you functioning longer.

Come learn about . . .

PREVENTING PARKINSON'S PROBLEMS

at:

_____

on:

_____

in:

_____

Taught by: _____

LISTEN, LEARN, AND EXERCISE!

PREVENTING PARKINSON'S PROBLEMS

Preventing Parkinson's Problems

LECTURE/DISCUSSION

In Parkinson's disease, there is a change in the transmitters in the nervous system. As a result, it is more difficult to initiate movements, and movements are very stiff. Classically, people with Parkinson's disease tend to shuffle, for example. These exercises are intended to help you relax, to loosen your muscles, to improve your posture, and to help you make the most of the muscle and nerve input that remains. It is important to do these on a regular basis. The most important thing to remember is to do as much of the activity as you can tolerate, but try not to tire yourself out completely. Remember to relax, breathe deeply, and let your body cooperate with you as much as possible. When walking, try to take steps as big as you are comfortable taking. We are going to go through and do the standing and sitting exercises, and we will talk about the ones to do on your stomach and back. Before you leave, I will give you a handout with these exercises on it so that you can do them at home.

EXERCISES

Sitting

1. Yardstick squeeze. Hold a yardstick with your hands wide apart on the stick. Bring it straight up over your head; then lower it behind your head (Figure 18-1). Squeeze your shoulder blades together. Relax. Repeat five times.
2. Yardstick tuck. Hold the yardstick with your hands close together. Bring it up behind your head. Pull your elbows back. Tuck your chin in, and push your neck back into the yardstick. Relax. Repeat five times.
3. Arm raises. While holding a can of soup or vegetables in your left hand,
   (a) and keeping your elbow straight, raise your arm straight up frontward. Lower and relax.
   (b) and keeping your elbow straight, raise your arm out to the side. Lower and relax.
   (c) put your hand behind your back. Slide it up your backbone as high as you can.
   (d) begin with your elbows bent, raise your arm straight up over your head.
   (e) with your arm at your side and your hand resting in your lap, bend your elbow.

Start by doing each exercise ten times. As you can, increase the number of repetitions to fifteen times. When fif-

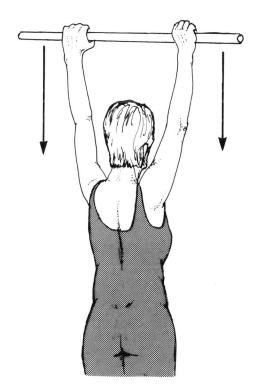 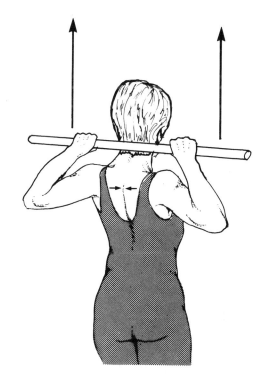

Figure 18-1 Lifting Yardstick and Squeezing Shoulders

teen times is easy, progress to using a heavier weight (a heavier can or other weight, about two to three pounds).

4. Palm push. Clasp your hands together so that your hands are up at the level of your neck or just below your neck. Push your palms together for a count of six.
5. Marches. While sitting, take "marching" steps. Alternately raise each leg from the chair, bringing your knee up toward the ceiling. Bring the knee up as *high* as you can each time. Repeat five times.
6. Knee straighteners. Sit with a rolled-up towel under each knee. Straighten the left knee, then the right. Straighten all the way. Progress to straightening your leg while the opposite leg is crossed over the one you are exercising. Repeat five times.
7. Ankle crosses. Cross your left leg over the right leg at the ankle. Try to bend the leg on top at the knee while you try to straighten the lower leg. Hold for a count of four. Relax. Switch so that the right leg is on top, and repeat the exercise. Repeat five times. Do exercises 5 through 7 ten times twice a day.
8. Table slide. Sit in a chair in front of a table. Clasp your hands together. Stretch your arms straight out in front of you on the table, and push your arms forward across the table and back toward your body along the table, using your whole body. Start with five times.
9. Table slide rock. Do a table slide, but rock forward far enough to lift your body out of the chair. Start with five times.

Do not sit for longer than a half hour at any one time. After half an hour, stand up at the chair, and do standing exercises.

Breathing Exercises

These breathing exercises are to be done lying on your back, sitting, and standing. *Do not* take more than five deep breaths in a row without resuming normal breathing.

1. Abdomen breaths. Put your hand on your abdomen. As you take a deep breath, push your hand out. Exhale through pursed lips. Repeat five times.
2. Lower rib breaths. Put your hands on the outside of your lower ribs. As you take a deep breath, push your ribs out toward your hands. Exhale through pursed lips. Repeat five times.
3. Upper rib breaths. Put your hands over your upper ribs. As you take a deep breath, push these ribs frontward toward your hands. Exhale through pursed lips. Repeat five times.
4. Diaphragmatic breathing: Breathe in through your nose and out through your mouth with your lips slightly closed. Make your expirations longer than your inspirations, but do not force air out. If you are using your diaphragm, you will feel movement under the rib cage and minimal chest movement. Breathe in, saying "my body is calm." Breathe out, saying "my body is quiet." Begin with three times per day, and gradually increase.

Facial Exercises

1. Chaw (exaggerated chewing), not chew, bubble gum for five minutes daily.
2. Say "ah-h-h-h," prolonging the sound for five seconds.
3. Grin, then pucker your lips.
4. Blow out, then suck in your cheek.
5. Pretend your tongue is cleaning food from between your cheek and teeth.
6. Speak or read with exaggerated mouth movements for short intervals several times daily.

7. Make faces at yourself in a mirror (Figure 18-2).

Exercises in the Prone Position

Lie on your stomach, and put one or two pillows under your abdomen.

1. With your arms straight above your head resting on the bed, raise your arms and shoulders up off the bed, and try to look at the ceiling. Hold for a count of three (Figure 18-3).
2. With your arms straight out to the side, raise your arms up off the bed. Hold for a count of three.
3. With your arms down by your side, lift them up off the bed. Hold for a count of three.

Do exercises 1 through 3 five times a day, and progress to ten times as you are able.

4. Keep your right knee straight. Raise the entire leg off the bed. Alternate with the left leg.
5. Bend your right knee. Now raise your right knee up off the bed as high as you can. Alternate with the left leg.

Repeat exercises 4 and 5 ten times each. Do not allow your body to roll to the side during this exercise.

Exercises in the Supine Position

1. Bring your right leg up to your chest as far as you can. Hold it there, and push your left leg down as if to stretch it and make it long. Repeat with the opposite leg.
2. With the right knee slightly bent, lift the right leg up off the bed as high as you can. You should feel a pull behind the knee. Alternate legs. Repeat ten times.
3. Spread your legs apart as far as you can. Then bring them back together. Repeat ten times.

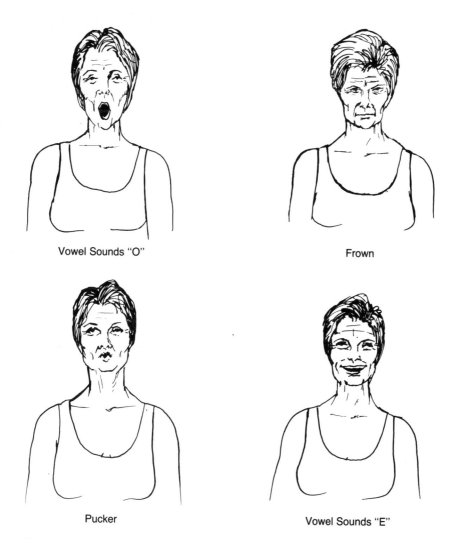

Vowel Sounds "O"   Frown

Pucker   Vowel Sounds "E"

Figure 18-2 Facial Exercises

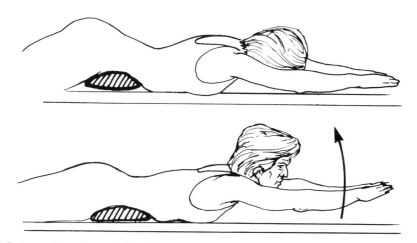

Figure 18-3 Lying on Your Stomach Stretch

4. Keep entire back flat on floor for five, ten, fifteen seconds.

Do the following exercises in the prone position with both knees and hips bent.

1. Raise your seat up off the bed. Repeat twenty times.
2. Try to do a sit-up. Repeat ten times.
3. Knee rolls. With your back and shoulders flat, your head on a pillow, your arms to the side, and your knees flexed with feet flat on the bed, rock your knees to the right and then to the left. Start with five to each side.
4. Head rocks. Lying in bed, gently rock your head side to side. Start with five times to each side. Increase to ten.

Standing

1. Shoulder shrugs: Bring shoulders around in big circles, three times clockwise and three times counterclockwise.
2. Chin tucks: Stand as erect as you can with your neck drawn back and your chin tucked in, not up. Do not tilt your chin. Pull your neck back in line with your spine, keeping your chin horizontal. Hold the position for ten seconds. Relax. Breathe. Repeat three times.
3. Hip circles. Make a circle with your hips without moving your shoulders. Start with five times in each direction. Increase to ten.

Opposing Osteoporosis

Osteoporosis is a disease in which the bones become thin. As a result, fractures can occur.

Did you know that certain exercises can help prevent further osteoporosis?

Come learn about . . .

OPPOSING OSTEOPOROSIS

at:

_____

on:

_____

in:

_____

Taught by: _____

LISTEN, LEARN, AND EXERCISE!

OPPOSING OSTEOPOROSIS

Opposing Osteoporosis

LECTURE/DISCUSSION

Osteoporosis is a disease in which the bones become thin and porous. As a result of this, fractures can occur.

Fractures are more common in women than in men. The disease is more commonly seen in whites than in blacks. There are three major sites for fractures: the hip, the spine, and the wrist.

One of the most common fractures is a hip fracture. A hip fracture is usually a fracture of the thigh bone or femur. It requires immediate medical attention. Patients are usually in the hospital for three to six weeks.

The bones of the spine (the vertebrae) are often the first to show signs of osteoporosis. The vertebrae may become thin and weak and ultimately fracture. The pain associated with spinal fractures has two phases. The acute phase, which is extreme, lasts one to four weeks; the chronic phase is bothersome and lasts six weeks. The osteoporosis victim with ver-

tebrae fracture has to contend with deformity, disability, and stress from the disease.

Osteoporosis can be detected, but usually extensive bone loss has occurred by the time it is diagnosed. Blood and urine tests can detect bone by-products. These tests show whether the body is using calcium or getting rid of it. Bone loss can also be detected with X-rays; however, by the time bone loss is detectable on an X-ray, the victim has lost at least 30 percent of his or her bone mass. Other detection methods are singular photon absorptiometry and computerized axial tomography (CAT) scan. These tests can detect bone loss early and even predict bone loss for young women.

Even without sophisticated tests or equipment, certain people can recognize if they are at high risk for osteoporosis. An allergy to milk or other dairy products indicates a susceptibility to osteoporosis. Problems with estrogen and/or progesterone levels are also common in those who will develop osteoporosis. Bone loss may become obvious in the person who is becoming shorter. Back pain and a change in posture could be signs of spinal fracture.

One of the most effective ways of treating osteoporosis seems to be taking estrogen

Source: Reprinted from *Osteoporosis Exercise Booklet*, Carole B. Lewis and Germaine Ferrall, an Aspen Consumer Information Pamphlet, © 1987 by Aspen Publishers, Inc.

on a short-term basis. Estrogen treatment prevents bone loss after removal of ovaries or during and after menopause. When menopause occurs, there is a drop in estrogen and a drop in bone buildup. Estrogen allows calcium to be more efficiently absorbed through the intestines. It also acts on the thyroid gland to produce calcitonin. Calcitonin, a hormone, protects bones from the dissolving effects of the parathyroid hormone. Estrogen also stimulates the liver to produce proteins that combine with adrenal hormones in the blood and prevent bone loss.

The problem with estrogen therapy is an increased risk of cancer; however, definitive research is forthcoming.

Calcium is another solution to the problem of osteoporosis. The daily calcium intake of the average period is about 400–500 milligrams per day. For postmenopausal women, calcium intake should be 1000 to 1500 milligrams per day. High intake of calcium reduces age-related bone loss and reduces fractures with osteoporosis patients. An increase in calcium intake should decrease the number of osteoporotic women. Calcium should be consumed whether a woman is on estrogen therapy or pursuing an exercise program. Consult your pharmacist regarding the type of calcium supplement best for you.

Research in osteoporosis led to an understanding of the effects of physical activity on bone mass. Lack of physical activity causes bone loss. Researchers have reported that bone converts mechanical energy to electrical energy. When negative charges were applied to bone tissue, there was a calcium buildup. When positive charges were applied to bone tissue, there was a calcium breakdown. These reactions can be reproduced naturally by the body. To receive a negative charge, stress must be applied to the bone tissue; the result is bone tissue buildup. The bone tissue not stressed receives a positive charge, and the result is bone breakdown. The major forces on bone are muscle contraction and gravity.

The more you stand, walk, and keep active, the better it is for your bones. Bones form in relationship to the stress put upon them. For example, when you lie down, your bones are not weight bearing (or stressed) so they will not be getting stronger. Sitting is better than lying down, standing is better than sitting, and walking is better than standing. Walking, housework, gardening, or caring for grandchildren are all activities that can help bones become stronger. Some suggested activities are:

Walking	Standing and
Standing and	cooking dinner
watering garden	Walking to the
Sweeping	mailbox
Grocery shopping	Walking to the bus
Walking with	Walking to a movie
grandchildren	Walking to the
Walking the dog	drugstore
	Standing at sink
	doing dishes

Today's exercise session contains weight-bearing exercises that are designed to help increase bone mass. A few postural exercises are also included to help improve forces on the bone and decrease the incidents of fractures. To be effective, these exercises should be done at least twice a day.

One point before we begin exercises. If you experience pain in your joints while doing the exercises or afterwards, do not continue. Consult your physical therapist or physician. First, I will show you the exercises. Then we will do them together. Then we will run through all the exercises to music. Before you leave today, I will give you a handout with these exercises and some helpful hints on opposing osteoporosis (*Appendix 19-A*).

EXERCISES: STRONGER BONE STROLL

1. Foot bone. Stand and grasp the chair back. Raise up on your toes, and then slowly return to the starting position. Repeat five times.

2. Shin bone. Keep grasping the chair back. Raise your leg toward the wall, and push the outside of your foot gently against the wall. Hold five seconds. Repeat five times each. (You may have to pretend there is a wall.)

3. Thigh bone. Still grasping the chair back, take ten slow steps in place. Repeat five times.

4. Hip bone. Still grasping the chair back, move your hips clockwise. Move your hips counterclockwise. Repeat five times. Now, let us sit down for the rest of the exercises.

5. Tail bone. Put your hands on the small of your back and arch backwards. Return to your normal sitting position. Repeat five times.

6. Back bone. With your hands on your shoulders, slowly sway from side to side. Slowly sway from front to back. Repeat five times.

7. Shoulder bone. With your hands at your sides, pull your shoulder blades together in back, and tuck in your chin. Hold five seconds. Relax. Repeat five times.

8. Arm bone. Place the palms of your hands on the wall or chair in front of you. Lean toward the wall with your body, keeping hands in place. Then push back away from the wall or chair to the starting position. (You may need to imagine a wall on this one.) Repeat five times.

9. Elbow bone. Slowly nod your head forward, and press your forehead against your right palm. Nod backward, and press the back of your head against the left palm. Nod from side to side, pressing sides of head against each palm. Repeat five times.

10. Finger bone. Touch both palms together and press gently against palms and fingers. Release. Repeat five times.

11. Sit back on your chair, and take three deep relaxing breaths.

You have just completed the Bone-to-Bone, Stronger Bone Stroll. Remember to do these exercises daily, and, most of all, enjoy! Now, let's go through the entire routine with music. Do the exercises 1 through 11 and then 11 through 1.

Appendix 19-A

Opposing Osteoporosis Handout

Hints

1. Do not stand or walk for such long periods that you begin to hurt or feel pain in your joints.
2. It is better to stand, walk, or sit for short, but frequent, periods.
3. Start your standing, sitting, or walking program for short periods, and build up your endurance. For example, a model activity program (standing, sitting, and walking) would be:

    Week 1: 5 minutes every hour
    Week 2: 10 minutes every hour
    Week 3: 15 minutes every hour
    Week 4: 20 minutes every hour

4. If an increase in activity starts to hurt, return to an easier level, and stay there two or three weeks, then try the more difficult level again.
5. If pain begins with the sitting, standing, or walking program

and persists for an hour after you have stopped the activity, contact your doctor or physical therapist.
6. Preplan your sitting, standing, or walking activities. For example, do not walk farther than you can safely return.
7. Most important, enjoy being more active and feeling stronger in your muscles and bones.

Do's

1. Complete your exercise program every day. Activity is essential.
2. Try to participate in a regular walking program, if your physical condition permits this.
3. Watch your posture. Be careful to sit and stand tall. Avoid sleeping in a curled position on your side.
4. Pick up all throw rugs, and make certain all carpet edges are securely fastened to the floor to avoid falls.
5. Try increasing the wattage of lighting in hallways, bathrooms,

and kitchen areas. Try a night-light near the bed to improve night safety.

6. Wear soft-heeled shoes and thick socks to decrease shock to the weight-bearing bones.

7. Use a cane or other walking aid if recommended. It can help relieve stress over weaker areas and increase your stability.

8. Use a "reacher" device to help avoid stooping to pick things off the floor. Try long-handled cleaning brushes and tools.

9. Increase your intake of calcium-rich foods, such as skim milk and spinach, or take calcium supplements. Discuss this with your doctor if you have any other medical condition that may be aggravated by extra calcium.

10. Notify your doctor immediately if you develop any sudden pain, swelling, or tenderness over any bone.

Don'ts

1. Do not take to your chair. Remain active. Inactivity is the worst thing for osteoporosis.
2. Do not despair. Your bones are alive and changing as long as you are.

Exercises: Stronger Bone Stroll

1. Foot bone: Repeat five times.
2. Shin bone: Repeat five times each.
3. Thigh bone: Repeat five times.
4. Hip bone: Repeat five times.
5. Tail bone: Repeat five times.
6. Back bone: Repeat five times.
7. Shoulder bone: Repeat five times.
8. Arm bone: Repeat five times.
9. Elbow bone: Repeat five times.
10. Finger bone: Repeat five times.
11. Sit back on your chair, and take three deep relaxing breaths.

Perfect Posture

Posture tells people a lot about you. Good posture also helps your body function better.

Posture exercises are easy to learn so join us to find out about . . .

PERFECT POSTURE

at:

_____

on:

_____

in:

_____

Taught by: _____

LISTEN, LEARN, AND EXERCISE!

PERFECT POSTURE

Perfect Posture

LECTURE/DISCUSSION

Posture tells people a lot about you. Posture affects how you look, obviously; standing with your head in a very forward position makes you look sort of unhappy and depressed, while standing in a very chin-tucked, upright position makes you much more attractive. Good posture can also enhance your musculoskeletal and your cardiopulmonary functioning. For example, try this: stick your head way forward as far as you can (*demonstrate*), take a deep breath, and blow it out. Now, sit back in your chair, pull your head up as high as you can, and take a nice deep breath. Notice that you can take a much bigger breath when your head is back in the chin tuck position. So, posture is extremely important not only for physical attractiveness, but also for physical functioning.

Good posture can be looked at from either the side or the front. From the side, if you have good posture, you can draw a straight line from your ear, shoulder, knee, and ankle. Take a look at my posture. Then stand up, and take a quick look at the posture of the other members of the class (*go around to all the participants, giving quick little hints to people if they have a forward head,*

rounded shoulders, or bend in their knees; try to be positive, but try to give good useful feedback).

You can assess posture from the front or the back, too. People often have asymmetries. One shoulder may be higher; one hip may be higher. Such an asymmetry may cause problems. There may be a tightness or soreness in the higher shoulder. A higher hip may cause tightness in the back area as well. So again, stand up, and let me take a look at your posture (*again, go around the room and give individual feedback*).

Good posture is also needed when you are sitting down. For this, you need to support yourself with the back of a chair, behind your low back and behind your upper back area. So let's all sit back with good posture (*watch the participants, and give feedback to them*).

Try and become aware of your posture, and know when your posture is good. Do not take posture for granted. You really need to work on posture all the time. Put dots around your house or apartment, and every time you see a dot think to yourself that you need to tuck your chin in or pull your shoulders back. I will give you a handout before you leave today with some other reminders (*Appendix 20-A; read aloud and discuss, if desired.*) Now we are going to go on to posture exercises.

EXERCISES

1. Deep breaths. Do three times.
2. Turtle. Push head forward in an exaggerated motion, then pull back. Do three times.
3. Chin tucks. Do three times.
4. Head motions. Do three times each.
   (a) Forward
   (b) Backward
   (c) Side to side
   (d) Over each shoulder
5. Shoulder shrugs. Do three times.
6. Shoulder circles. Do three times.
7. Shoulder backs. Pull your shoulder blades back. Do three times.
8. Arm reaches up. Reach as high as you can to the sky. Do three times.
9. Arm reaches back. Reach as far backward as possible. Do three times.
10. Side tilts. Do three times.
11. Pelvic tucks. Do three times.
12. Gluteal sets. Tighten your buttock muscles as tight as you can. Do three times.
13. Knee ups. Bend your knees up to the ceiling. Alternate knees. Do three times.
14. Knee outs. Let your knees flop outward. Do three times.
15. Knee twists. Turn your knees inward. Do three times.
16. Ankle bends. Do three times.
17. Ankle circles. Do three times.
18. Toe curls. Do five times.
19. Spine lengtheners. As you take a deep breath, imagine your spine extending from your hips to the top of your head. Do three times.
20. Body extenders. Gently pull your spine into extension. Do three times.

Appendix 20-A

Perfect Posture Handout

Do's

1. Tuck in your chin.
2. Pull your shoulders back as much as you can.
3. Try to keep your ear over your shoulders, over your hips, over your ankles.
4. When sitting, support your back and legs as much as possible.
5. Think lengthening.
6. Try to sleep in a position that optimizes good posture and flexibility of muscles.
7. Be aware of your posture as much as possible.

Don'ts

1. Do not sit in one position too long.
2. Do not stand in one position too long.

Exercises

1. Deep breaths: Do three times.
2. Turtle: Do three times.
3. Chin tucks: Do three times.
4. Head motions: Do three times each.
   a. Forward
   b. Backward
   c. Side to side
   d. Over each shoulder
5. Shoulder shrugs: Do three times.

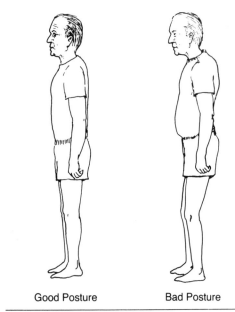

Good Posture   Bad Posture

6. Shoulder circles: Do three times.
7. Shoulder backs: Do three times.
8. Arm reaches up: Do three times.
9. Arm reaches back: Do three times.
10. Side tilts: Do three times.
11. Pelvic tucks: Do three times.
12. Gluteal sets: Do three times.
13. Knee ups: Do three times.
14. Knee outs: Do three times.
15. Knee twists: Do three times.
16. Ankle bends: Do three times.
17. Ankle circles: Do three times.
18. Toe curls: Do five times.
19. Spine lengtheners: Do three times.
20. Body extenders: Do three times.

21

Getting Stronger

As you get older, you need to work on your strength so that you can continue all your activities.

Learn the correct strengthening exercises at the class on . . .

GETTING STRONGER

at:

_____

on:

_____

in:

_____

Taught by: _____

LISTEN, LEARN, AND EXERCISE!

GETTING STRONGER

21

Getting Stronger

LECTURE/DISCUSSION

As we grow older, we are faced with decisions. We know, for example, that muscles become lax if we do not use them. This is where the "use it or lose it" principle arises. Muscle cells cannot regenerate; therefore, when cells die, they are not replaced. If we do not take care of the remaining muscles, they can also waste away from disuse.

There are three kinds of muscles in our bodies: cardiac muscle, smooth muscle, and skeletal muscle. Cardiac muscle is found only in the heart, and its primary function is to keep the heart pumping. Smooth muscle is found in many different places and has a variety of functions. For example, smooth muscles line the blood vessels, dilate your eye pupils, and help to move waste products through the intestines. Skeletal muscle, which is literally attached to the bones by tendons and connective tissue, has the sole purpose of moving body parts.

There are more than 600 muscles in the body. Some are small, like the muscles in the hands, while some are big, like the ones in the thighs. As we get older, we lose strength in our smaller muscles first. Not all loss of strength is due to age or size of the muscle, however. For example, people who have remained sedentary most of their lives, have eaten poorly, or suffer from poor innervation to certain muscles can expect a certain amount of atrophy, that is, wasting away, of the muscles. Certain diseases, such as muscular dystrophy and multiple sclerosis, also cause muscle weakness.

What kinds of movements build muscle strength? Basically, three kinds of contractions build muscle strength: isometric, isotonic, and isokinetic. For the most part, isometric contractions are not favored for individuals who are fifty years of age and older. Why? In an isometric contraction, there is no pressure at the joint; there is only internal pressure in the muscle. For example, clench your fist. When some of you did that, you held your breath. When you force a contraction and hold your breath, you can elevate your blood pressure rather suddenly, causing injury. Moreover, because there is no movement of the joint, there is no benefit in terms of flexibility. Exercises that do not enhance flexibility while building strength are inadequate as a sole source of activity.

On the other hand, an all-around exercise that is isotonic, such as walking, bicycle riding, or low-impact aerobics, is great for the body. Isotonic exercises, by definition, involve the full range of motion for the joints and build strength. This is the most recommended form of exercise for any individual.

Isokinetic exercises develop maximum tension in a muscle throughout the entire range of motion, but they require special equipment. Therefore, we will not pursue this discussion. Isokinetic exercises are good for older adults who are being monitored as they work, however.

Strength is built by training, that is, repeated performances. How often you should go through a strength-building exercise routine depends on what you want to accomplish. Three times a week should be the minimum. You may prefer to break up your exercise routines into two days for the upper body and three days for the lower body, however. You should exercise anywhere from 20 to 30 minutes. Do not exhaust yourself. That is why breaking a routine into separate routines to work on different muscle groups is a good idea (i.e., upper body one day and lower body the next). It is important to tire the muscle to benefit in strength gains, though. Usually, people do three sets of ten repetitions with weights. If you are doing calisthenics and not using weights, however, the number of repetitions for each exercise varies.

Using weights is contraindicated for some individuals, such as those with cardiac disease or hypertension, so obtaining a doctor's approval is important if you fall within these categories. Depending on your physical condition and your doctor's advice, you may want to start with small weights. A two-pound weight for biceps curls or other arm exercises may be just enough. Home-made devices, such as one-quart milk cartons filled with water or tins half-filled with sand, are also useful. A device for leg lifts can be made from two old socks, with a full tin can in each, sewn or tied together. This device fits easily over your ankle and is affordable (*demonstrate*).

All exercises, if done on a consistent and regular basis, build strength. Extra weight, such as heavy books or plastic pint, quart, or gallon jugs filled with water in the hands, can be used in exercises for each body part to increase strength. Remember to breathe in before exertion and out while exerting any force. Never hold your breath.

In order to gauge how much weight you can lift, see if you can do the exercise with a minimal weight for ten repetitions. That will equal one set. If you can do the exercise, try another set. Work up to three sets.

You do not need to use weights in order to gain strength to maintain everyday functioning. If you would like to use weights, however, think about these beginner's tips.

- Follow a system. A system is developed by repeating an exercise four to ten times. For example, you would do four repetitions of a biceps curl, rest for about one minute, then do four more repetitions, rest for about one minute, and do four more again.
- When you have completed three sets of four repetitions, you are ready to go on to another exercise.
- Your weight should be heavy enough for you to complete about eight to ten repetitions. If you cannot do at least eight, your weight is too heavy and needs to be decreased.
- If you begin to lift weights, you must make a commitment to do it at least three times a week, or else you will gain little benefit and risk tremendous injury.

I will give you a handout before you leave today with some tips on getting stronger (*Appendix 21-A; read aloud and discuss if desired*).

EXERCISES

1. Postural check.
2. Warm-up exercises (see Chapter 4, class routine).

BIBLIOGRAPHY

Fitness, Health & Nutrition. Alexandria, Va.: Time-Life Books, Inc., 1987.

Getting Firm. Alexandria, Va.: Time-Life Books, Inc., 1987.

Overton, Ted. *Sports after Fifty.* Annapolis, Md.: Azimuth Press, Inc., 1988.

Appendix 21-A

Getting Stronger Handout

Hints

1. Get the permission of your doctor to start a strength-building program if you have a heart condition, high blood pressure, or detached retinas.
2. Never try to impress someone by overdoing an exercise. You will be foolishly risking injury.
3. Breathe evenly and steadily. Holding your breath can prevent blood from returning to your heart.
4. Rest between exercises if you are tired.
5. Make sure you are not hyperextending your wrist when using hand weights. Keep your hand aligned with your arm to prevent damage to the wrist.

Do's

1. Warm up for ten minutes before starting any exercise regimen.
2. Cool down when you finish an exercise regimen. If you suddenly stop what you are doing without cooling down, blood will pool in your legs, causing a sudden drop in blood pressure that could result in fainting.
3. Use controlled movements when you exercise. You will be conserving energy in the long run, as well as decreasing risk of injury to joints and muscles.
4. Work larger muscle groups first. That way you are using this time as an additional warm-up for the rest of the body.

Don'ts

1. Do not lift any weight if you have a lower back problem or are recovering from surgery.
2. Do not exercise on a hard floor. You can injure your joints or spine.
3. Do not exercise every day. Your body needs a chance to rest.
4. Do not ever do straight-legged sit-ups for abdominal strength. Always bend your knees, make sure your lower back is flat on the floor (pelvic tilt), and only come

up six inches from the floor with your shoulders. If you sit up all the way, you are exercising a different set of muscle groups. Also, keep your stomach muscles tightened to enhance the exercise. Keep your chin slightly tucked to prevent neck strain. A tuck that is too tight, however, will prevent normal blood flow to the head. Think of an orange under the chin.

5. Do not grip hand weights too tightly. This increases internal pressure, which, in turn, increases blood pressure. It also puts excessive pressure on the fragile joints of the fingers.

Exercises

1. Postural check

2. Warm-up exercises
   - deep breaths
   - chin tucks
   - shoulder rolls
   - arm stretches
   - side reaches
   - leg strengtheners
   - ankle bends
   - toe curls
   - ankle circles

3. Biceps curl
4. Bottom tighteners
5. Inner leg press
6. Outer leg press
7. Back kicks
8. Shoulder presses
9. Pelvic tilts
10. Sit-ups

Better Breathing

Don't take your breathing for granted. You can feel better just by breathing better.

Learn more about breathing at the class on . . .

BETTER BREATHING

at:

_____

on:

_____

in:

_____

Taught by: _____

LISTEN, LEARN, AND EXERCISE!

BETTER BREATHING

Better Breathing

LECTURE/DISCUSSION

Sometimes when you feel tired, concerned about something, or worried about a task you perceive to be difficult, you sigh. Some people have speculated that such a sigh is a subconscious action in response to the body's need for a moment of relaxation, a moment to initiate the calming and soothing effect of a full deep breath.

Unless something impairs it or it fails us, we generally take breathing for granted. Many people have some impairment of their breathing system, however. Many of you here may suffer from asthma, emphysema, or some other respiratory disease (*ask if anyone has a breathing impairment, what type it is, and if he or she is taking any medication*). To find out what kind of breathing you use most often—shallow breathing, deep breathing, or a combination of the two—place the palm of your left hand flat in the middle of your chest. Your fingers should be fanned out so that your pinky is resting right at the top of your diaphragm, like this (*demonstrate*). Now, place the pinky finger of your right hand at your bellybutton, and rest the palm of your hand comfortably on your stomach (*demonstrate*).

Just relax, breathe as you normally do, and think about the following questions: Is your right hand moving? Is your left hand moving? Are both hands moving? If only your left hand is moving, you are breathing shallow breaths. If only your right hand is moving, you are breathing deep breaths. If both hands are moving, you have a combination of both types of breathing.

Deep breathing is best because, as we get older, the lower lobes of the lungs do not receive as much oxygen as they did when we were younger. Shallow breathing ultimately places more work on the heart, because you must take more breaths in order to obtain an adequate amount of oxygen. It is important to maximize the amount of oxygen getting to the muscles and the surrounding tissue, as well as to the brain. Unfortunately, most people do not breathe deeply, even though it is a very natural way. For example, think about a newborn baby. The baby's stomach is distended when air is inhaled, and it retracts when air is exhaled. That is the way people were meant to breathe.

We need about 2,300 gallons of air every day. A person who is thirty years old breathes about 135 gallons of air each hour.

A person who is over sixty-five years old breathes about 95 gallons of air each hour. That amounts to approximately 1,000 gallons less each day. In order to increase the amount of air we breathe, it is necessary first to strengthen our chest and back muscles. Strengthening and retraining the muscles in the diaphragm and the abdomen are also important for effective breathing. They help pull out your chest and stomach at inhalation and help to push out the air at exhalation. Second, we need to practice controlled breathing, because slower and deeper breathing will probably make you feel more energetic. Your mind will become more alert, and the lower lobes of your lungs will get the ventilation that has been missing. Basically, air flows into the lungs when many parts of the respiratory system function together. For example, the diaphragm pulls downward to create more volume, the chest walls expand outward, and the clavicles (collar bones) move upward. This is a simple description of a very complex mechanism.

The best way to ensure that the tissues are getting enough oxygen is to employ diaphragmatic breathing. The lower lobes (bottom third) of the lungs are best reached through this type of breathing. Also, as the diaphragm contracts, it pushes the abdominal organs forward and down. This rhythmical, internal massage gently squeezes the abdominal organs, enhancing circulation. Diaphragmatic breathing also increases vital capacity, that is, the amount of air that we can breathe in, and helps to empty our lungs more efficiently. This latter function is especially important for older people, as more stale air is left in the lungs as we get older. Diaphragmatic breathing also reduces strain on the heart by decreasing the number of breaths that you must take per minute and strengthens the muscles involved in the breathing process. As an added benefit, it relaxes the body by reducing anxiety. Take some time now to practice diaphragmatic breathing.

Before you leave today, I will give you a handout with some do's and don'ts for better breathing (*Appendix 22-A; read aloud and discuss, if desired*).

EXERCISES

Postural check. Poor posture weakens the back and abdominal muscles. If you are seated for a prolonged amount of time with no change in position to correct slouching or improper neck positions, you are adding to poor breathing habits. Therefore, it is important to check your posture before doing breathing exercises.

1. Nose breathing. Always remember to breathe in and out through your nose. For those of you who are not used to it, try it as you breathe normally.
2. Inhalation process. As you are sitting up straight and comfortably, move up in your chair so that your body does not touch the back of your chair. Place both hands on your stomach, fanning out your fingers to cover as much of the area as possible.
   (a) Exhale the last breath you took (Figure 22-1).
   (b) As you begin to inhale, relax your stomach muscles, and feel your hands move outward as your belly extends.
   (c) Now, keep filling up your chest cavity so that your chest and rib cage expand.
   (d) As you progress, you will feel the top of your chest and your collar bones rise. Keep your belly out, even though you are tempted to pull it in.
   (e) Exhale as you normally would, and take a couple of regular breaths so that you do not feel uncomfortable. The process of inhaling correctly will probably take you about six seconds. Within four to six weeks, if you practice this daily for about five minutes, the inhalation process may take as long as ten or twelve seconds.

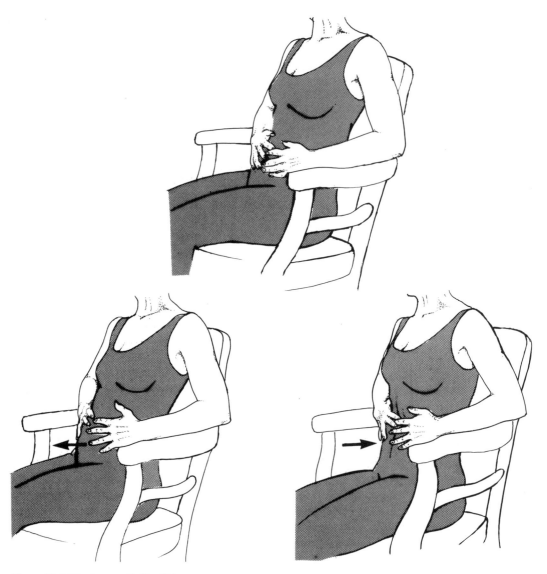

Figure 22-1 Diaphragmatic Breathing

3. Exhalation process. Repeat the inhalation exercise, and add the exhalation process.
   (a) After inhaling to the best of your ability, hold your breath for a second; then begin to exhale as slowly as possible. Do not expel the air in one big burst. Control your breathing.
   (b) As you exhale, your hands on your stomach should move inward.
   (c) Repeat the whole breathing process again, focusing on control and movement of the diaphragm.
   (d) At the end of the exhalation process, you may pull your stomach in slightly to force all of the air out.

Once you have the rhythm correct and understand that the stomach fills out with inhalation and tucks in with exhalation, you should remove your hands when doing these exercises.

Appendix 22-A

Better Breathing Handout

Do's

1. Practice your breathing exercises every day for three to five minutes, morning and evening.
2. Place your hands on your stomach to determine whether you are breathing correctly.
3. Breathe slowly and rhythmically.
4. Wear comfortable clothes to encourage proper breathing.

Don'ts

1. Do not breathe so deeply that you exhaust yourself or become dizzy. This is an indication that you are not breathing normally.
2. Do not smoke cigarettes, cigars, or smokeless cigarettes.

3. Do not attempt to do deep breathing exercises outdoors when the pollen count is high if you have allergies.
4. Do not expand the chest first when you inhale. Remember, the belly pushes out first, not the chest.

Exercises

1. Postural check
2. Nose breaths
3. Inhalation process
4. Exhalation process

Note: Repeat these exercises every day while sitting quietly or just before taking a nap or retiring for the evening.

Stopping Stroke

A stroke can be very debilitating. However, a home exercise program can keep you functioning longer.

Come learn about these exercises for . . .

STOPPING STROKE

at:

_____

on:

_____

in:

_____

Taught by: _____

LISTEN, LEARN, AND EXERCISE!

STOPPING STROKE

23

Stopping Stroke

LECTURE/DISCUSSION

A stroke is basically a stoppage of blood to the brain. It can result from an embolus, which is a tiny blood clot that travels through the vessels in the brain and stops the blood from getting to parts of the brain; a thrombus, which is an accumulation of plaque that blocks the blood vessels and prevents blood from getting to parts of the brain; or a hemorrhage, a condition in which blood begins to seep out of the blood vessels of the brain. Whatever the cause, the person does not get enough blood to a particular area of the brain, and the opposite side of the body is affected. For example, if the stroke happens on the right side of the brain, the person will have problems on the left side of the body. Problems range from a totally spastic arm or leg to an inability to move the involved side of the body. Spasticity may have a peculiar pattern. The person may try to lift an arm, but cannot lift the arm in a straightforward manner; instead, the person lifts the arm in a tight, very toned pattern (*demonstrate*). Or, the person may try to step with the toes pointed very straight (*demonstrate*).

As patients progress through a stroke rehabilitation program, they may be able eventually to change their movement pat-

terns. They may go from a flaccid position (or no movement position) to a spastic position to a normal position. Not everybody recovers from a stroke to the same extent or at the same pace. Whatever the problem, it is a good idea to keep the involved side moving as normally as possible and to keep it strong and flexible. People have been known to recover from a stroke even a year after the stroke occurred, so it is important to continue to exercise. I have a handout with helpful hints for stopping stroke that I will give you before you leave today (*Appendix 23-A; read aloud and discuss, if desired*).

The program that we are going to do is motion exercises, warm-up, standing exercises, and deep breathing. The other thing that I would like to encourage you to do at home is bike riding or any activity that stimulates your cardiovascular system.

EXERCISES

1. Sitting shoulder cradle. Cradle your elbow in your hand. Bring your elbow up in the air three times. Bring your elbow out to the side three times. You can passively move your weaker arm or use it to help as much as possible.

130

2. Arm turns. Hold your arm at the wrist and turn the arm out (sitting sideways in the chair). Repeat five times.
3. Wrist grasps. Touch your shoulder and pull your arm down between your legs. Turn the palm up and down. Repeat three times.
4. Hand grasps. Bend your hand up and down. Repeat three times.
5. Finger bends. Bend your fingers up and down. Repeat three times.
6. Standing toe ups. Standing, go up and down on your toes. Repeat five times.
7. Leg raises to the side. Raise your leg out to the right side, then to the left side. Repeat five times.
8. Leg raises. Raise your leg to the front, then to the right and left. Repeat five times.
9. Leg kicks. Kick your leg to the back, to the right, and then to the left. Repeat five times.
10. Heel walks. Walk ten steps on your heels.
11. Side walks. Walk ten steps sideways.
12. Back walks. Walk ten steps backward.
13. Sitting shoulder shrugs. Sit and do five shoulder shrugs.
14. Ankle bends. Bend your ankles up and down. Repeat five times.
15. Ankle circles. Make circles with your ankles. Repeat five times.
16. Ankle turns. Turn your ankles in and out. Repeat five times.
17. Leg kicks. Do leg kicks in the air. Repeat five times.
18. Leg aparts. Bring your legs apart and together in the air. Repeat five times.

Appendix 23-A

Stopping Stroke Handout

Hints

1. Never give up. Always remember that there are some things that you can try to do to improve your functional status.
2. Try to adapt your environment to help you live independently.
3. There is no cure; hard work is the only answer.
4. Try to accept your limitations and work within them.

Do's

1. Try to find comfortable positions for sitting, standing, and walking.
2. Try to move around as much as possible.
3. Try to do as many activities as you can without discomfort.
4. Try as much as possible to relax your body.

Don'ts

1. Never maintain positions that cause you pain.
2. Do not fight with yourself to do activities.
3. Do not pull your involved extremities into positions that they do not want to be in.

4. Do not go for the quick cures. It is going to take hard work to make maximum use of your remaining functional abilities.

Exercises

1. Sitting shoulder cradle: Repeat three times.
2. Arm turns: Repeat five times.
3. Wrist grasps: Repeat three times.
4. Hand grasps: Repeat three times.
5. Finger bends: Repeat three times.
6. Standing toe ups: Repeat five times.
7. Leg raises to the side: Repeat five times.
8. Leg raises: Repeat five times.
9. Leg kicks: Repeat five times.
10. Heel walks: Walk on heels ten steps.
11. Side walks: Walk sideways ten steps.
12. Back walks: Walk backward ten steps.
13. Sitting shoulder shrugs: Repeat five times.
14. Ankle bends: Repeat five times.
15. Ankle circles: Repeat five times.
16. Ankle turns: Repeat five times.
17. Leg kicks: Repeat five times.
18. Leg aparts: Repeat five times.

Ways To Walk

More efficient walking can save you energy and time.

Please come and learn why and how to improve your . . .

WAYS TO WALK

at:

_____

on:

_____

in:

_____

Taught by: _____

LISTEN, LEARN, AND EXERCISE!

WAYS TO WALK

24

Ways To Walk

LECTURE/DISCUSSION

Today we are going to discuss ways to walk. When you walk, you are using momentum to the best of your ability. Basically, walking is a loss and recovery of balance and the use of momentum (*walk back and forth with a nice swing through*). As you walk, you are falling off one foot and catching yourself on the other. As you sit too long, you get weaker, and it becomes a little more difficult for you to walk.

A good gait has a swing-through phase, a weight-bearing phase, a push-off phase, and a heel strike phase. So, as you walk, you want to put down your heel, go on to your toe, and push off. Then just catch yourself on your other foot again (*demonstrate*). When we use momentum less, we tend to spend longer in the stance phase (*demonstrate, spending longer in the stance phase*). We are going to do some exercises that will increase your strength, and that will help you propel yourself as you walk along. I am going to give you a handout that will help you to remember what we talk about (Appendix 24-A; *read aloud and discuss, if desired*).

EXERCISES

Sitting

1. Toe ups. Sitting in your chair, go up and down on your toes. Repeat five times.
2. Heel rocks. Rock back onto your heels while you are sitting. This exercise is good for heel strike and push-off. Do this five times.
3. Leg straighteners. Straighten your legs out, and hold them in the air. Hold this position for ten seconds, and relax. Repeat five times.
4. Hip rocks. Rock your hips back and forth. Just roll your hips back and forth. Do this five times.
5. Shoulder rocks. Rock your shoulders back and forth. Rotate your trunk, and move your hips back and forth. Repeat five times.

Now you are ready to stand up and put some of these exercises into the gait pattern.

Standing

6. Standing toe ups. While standing and holding onto the back of a chair, go up on your toes. Repeat ten times.
7. Standing heel rocks. Rock back on your heels as far as you can. Repeat ten times.
8. Leg swings. While holding onto your chair, swing your foot out as far as you can. Repeat five times.
9. Back and forth leg swings. Swing your whole leg forward and backward. Repeat ten times.
10. Leg swing steps. Swing your leg back as far as you can; then swing it forward and step on it. Then rock back, swing your leg back again, and step on your heel. Do that four times on each leg.
11. Hip circles. Rock your hips around and around in a circle. Do three times one way, then three times the other.
12. Shoulder rolls. Roll your shoulders back and forth, left and right. Repeat five times.
13. Arm swings. While standing, swing your arms, from the sockets, forward and backward as far as you can. Repeat five times.
14. Calf stretches. Hold onto the chair, keep your heel back, and stretch the calf muscles as far as you can. Repeat five times.
15. Leg swing, heel hit. Hold onto your chair, swing your leg forward, hit your heel, land on it, bring your weight over your knee, and bend it just a little bit. Come back up, rock back, forward, rock back. Repeat three times with each leg.
16. Leg balance. Balance on each leg, arm in front of you. Try not to hold on, and see how long you can balance on each leg. Repeat three times.
17. Balance toe ups. Balance on each leg, and try to go up on your toes. Repeat five times.

Any time that you are walking, try these exercises, and see if you can improve your gait (*if you have time, evaluate each person's gait, and recommend specific exercises*).

Appendix 24-A

Ways To Walk Handout

Hints

1. Try to avoid sitting for long periods of time.
2. Find a safe place where you can walk and feel comfortable about not losing your balance, and practice taking longer steps. Practice swinging your leg out farther.
3. Try rotating your hips and shoulders a little more to get a little extra momentum.

Exercises

1. Toe ups: Repeat five times.
2. Heel rocks: Do this five times.
3. Leg straighteners: Repeat five times.
4. Hip rocks: Do this five times.
5. Shoulder rocks: Repeat five times.
6. Standing toe ups: Repeat ten times.
7. Standing heel rocks: Repeat ten times.
8. Leg swings: Repeat five times.
9. Back and forth leg swings: Repeat ten times.
10. Leg swing steps: Do this four times on each leg.

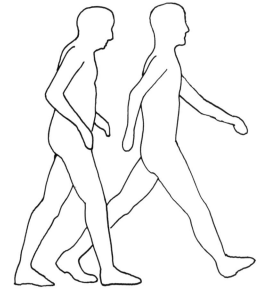

Older Walking Pattern   Younger Walking Pattern

11. Hip circles: Do three times one way, then three times the other.
12. Shoulder rolls: Repeat five times.
13. Arm swings: Repeat five times.
14. Calf stretches: Do this five times.
15. Leg swing, heel hit: Repeat three times with each leg.
16. Leg balance: Repeat three times with each leg.
17. Balance toe ups: Repeat five times.

25

Facts on Flexibility

Did you know that toe touches are *not* the true test of flexibility? Learn the

FACTS ON FLEXIBILITY

at:

_____

on:

_____

in:

_____

Taught by: _____

LISTEN, LEARN, AND EXERCISE!

FACTS ON FLEXIBILITY

Facts on Flexibility

LECTURE/DISCUSSION

Many people grew up thinking that toe touching was the bona fide test for flexibility. Actually, they are not altogether wrong—or right. Today, it is known that touching the toes indicates only the flexibility in the hamstrings (the muscles in the back of your upper thighs) and in the lower back. In fact, some people believe that, in certain circumstances, toe touching may be injurious to the body.

Flexibility is a term that describes the condition of the whole body. One rule of thumb is, never force or overstretch a muscle, because overdoing a stretch can lengthen ligaments as well as muscles. Remember that muscles extend and are elastic. Ligaments, the tissues that hold muscles to bones, are extensible, but not elastic; whereas muscles bounce back, ligaments stay stretched. For women who continued to wear very high heeled shoes over the years, for example, walking barefoot or wearing lower heeled shoes or slippers became both uncomfortable and painful. The ligaments became so overstretched that normal activity in different shoes was no longer possible.

It is never too late to become flexible, even with limited range of motion in the joints. Inflexibility can be reversed and joint stiffness can be slowly alleviated. Some people have backaches or unnecessary leg cramps at night. Both stretching and proper posture can help to strengthen the lower back and pelvic muscles, because it keeps pressure off the lower disc in the lumbar (lower back) area. So, regardless of age, anyone can improve flexibility. The advantage of maintaining flexibility is, ultimately, being able to move about while carrying on daily routines and having that extra safeguard of keeping the joints in good working condition.

A person who sits a great deal during the day is likely to feel tension build throughout the day in the neck, the shoulders, the lower back, and, perhaps, the buttocks. A person who stands for prolonged periods of time during the day may have aching feet and calves. Stretching any of these body parts helps to ease the tension produced in these muscle groups.

When they wake up in the morning, most people stretch very gently, slowly, and deliberately. That is exactly the right way to stretch: slowly and passively. Bouncing while stretching increases the risk of injury. A most effective way to stretch is to use an external force to help. For example, one or more limbs may be used for leverage to stretch another. Try flexing the fingers of your left hand backward. Now, use your right hand to help you with the stretch. This time, the stretch is quite different! Gravity can play an important role in stretching, too. For example, if you stand glued to the floor and slowly lean into a wall or door with both hands bracing yourself, the calf muscles in your lower leg will feel the stretch. That is gravity working with your body.

Sometimes when you are stretching a muscle, you may feel a twitch or contraction in another part of your body. Usually, this is the opposing muscle. For example, when the biceps is stretched, the triceps may be felt contracting. That is normal when starting a new stretching program. Eventually, you will gain control, and your stretches will feel "just right."

Before you leave today, I will give you some hints that will make everyday stretching easier and more productive (*Appendix 25-A; read aloud and discuss, if desired*).

EXERCISES

For each of the following exercises, hold the stretch for 15 seconds, and repeat each exercise at least five times. You are aiming for a stretch that is 10 percent beyond the normal length of the muscle.

1. Neck stretches. Place your right hand behind your head. Slowly, pull your head forward and to the right. Hold this stretch at a comfortable level for 15 seconds. You should feel this stretch in your neck and shoulder. Repeat, using your left hand and pulling your head to the left.
2. Shoulder/triceps stretches. Sit up straight, with your shoulders comfortably pulled back. Place your right palm behind your neck. Now, put your left hand on your right elbow, and pull your elbow toward the back of your head. You will be stretching the triceps in your right arm. Repeat, using your right hand to stretch your left arm triceps.
3. Cross body arm stretches. Place your right arm across your chest. Place your left hand on your elbow, and gently pull your right arm toward your left shoulder. This exercise enhances the stretch of the right triceps and shoulder. Repeat, using your left arm across the body and your right hand to pull (Figure 25-1).
4. Upper body twists. Sitting upright with both feet firmly planted on the floor, twist your upper torso to the left and hold onto the back of the chair with the right hand. (This exercise must be done cautiously when chairs have arm rests). Your left arm has come across your body to pull your upper and middle back muscles. Meanwhile, your right arm is holding onto the chair arm. Do not strain, but concentrate on using one continuous pull. Repeat to the opposite side of the body.
5. Open chest stretches. Sitting upright with your legs spread apart, reach with your left hand to grasp your left calf (if you cannot reach your calf, the knee is a good fixed point for beginners). Now, reach your right hand up into the air, opening your chest and elongating the muscles in your upper and middle back. Your head should also be turned to the right, while you gaze at your fingertips. Repeat once more, and do the exercise to the opposite side of the body.
6. Million dollar stretches. Place both arms above your head. Pretend that a check for one million dollars hangs directly above your head. Reach for the million, using alternate arm, side, and hand stretches. Do not stretch both arms at once. Use slow, deliberate reaches, stretching one arm up and then the other. Each arm should effect a stretch on the same side of the body, notably in the upper body.

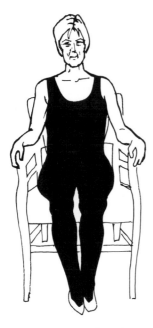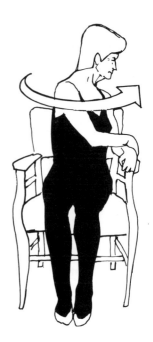

Figure 25-1 Cross Body Arm Stretch

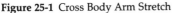

7. Calf stretches. Place the palms of your hands against the wall. Step forward with your left leg. Your right leg is locked at the knee while your left leg is forward and bent at the knee. You want to keep your right heel on the ground, since you are trying to stretch the gastrocnemius muscle, the muscle in your calf. Repeat, stretching the opposite calf.

8. Soleus stretches. In order to stretch the muscle that works in tandem with the gastrocnemius muscle, the soleus muscle, again place your palms against the wall with your left leg forward, and keep your right leg straight. Now, bend your right knee ever so slightly. Repeat, stretching the soleus muscle in the other leg. A good distance from the wall is considered arms' length.

9. Double calf stretches. Lean into the wall with both legs straight, knees locked, and heels flat on the floor. You should feel a stretch in your left and right gastrocnemius muscles.

10. Double soleus stretches. Again, lean into the wall. Bend at the knees slightly to stretch the left and right soleus muscles.

11. Foot sequences. Be seated comfortably. Using your right foot, point (extend) your toes as much as you can. Hold that position for 15 seconds. Turn your foot inward, and hold that stretch. Now, pull your toes up toward your shin bone, holding that stretch. Finally, turn your foot out, lengthening your inside of the foot muscle. Repeat this entire sequence at least one more time. Repeat with the left foot.

12. Total body stretch. Stand up. If you need assistance for balance, step behind your chair, and hold onto it. Stand up tall with your feet shoulder width apart and knees slightly bent. Reach up with your left arm while your right arm is relaxed in front of your pelvis. Continue your arm reach in a circular fashion so that you complete a semicircle, dropping

your left arm. When you come to the center, stand tall again, this time stretching your right arm in a semi-circle. As you return to center while doing this exercise, make sure that you feel the stretch in your waist. Now stand on your toes, and reach upward with your arms. Feel your body elongate; then slowly relax.

Appendix 25-A

Facts on Flexibility Handout

Hints

1. Always be aware of your posture. Good posture, whether sitting or standing, relaxes those muscle groups not needed to maintain your position and strengthens those that need it.
2. Take breaks during the day to stretch different body parts. It takes only a minute; it will energize you and help you to stay in tune with your body.
3. If you suffer from arthritis pain, take your medication to alleviate the pain before you begin to stretch. This allows you to stretch pain-free.
4. Take a hot bath or shower (water temperature at least 109 degrees) before beginning your stretches. It will increase the range of motion in your hip joint by 5 percent and will help relax your body.

Do's

1. Warm up the muscles that you will be stretching by doing slow, controlled movements that contract and relax those muscles.
2. Stretch every day at a time when you are not likely to be disturbed. Interruptions deter the progress you are making and may make it necessary to start all over again, including a warm-up.
3. Stretch slowly and progress slowly. You cannot force your body to be flexible overnight.
4. Wear comfortable, loose-fitting clothes with little or no jewelry.
5. Stretch different muscle groups for different reasons. The muscles that are the least flexible need to be stretched most often.
6. Test your flexibility periodically to see how well you are progressing.

Don'ts

1. Do not bounce when stretching; rather, stretch slowly and deliberately.
2. Do not stretch when you are too tired, in pain, or generally not

feeling well. Sloppy stretches lead to injury.

3. Do not take short, shallow breaths while stretching. Deep, slow breathing enhances movements and relaxes you.

4. Do not stretch after a meal. Your muscles will be competing with the digestion process for your blood supply.

5. Do not stretch fewer than three times a week. Any less will not improve flexibility.

6. Do not hold a stretch less than ten seconds.

7. Do not stretch to the point where you feel pain. If you do feel pain, stop and relax the stretch a bit until it feels better.

Exercises

1. Neck stretches: Repeat five times to each side.

2. Shoulder/triceps stretches: Repeat five times with each arm.

3. Cross body arm stretches: Repeat five times with each arm.

4. Upper body twists: Repeat five times to each side.

5. Open chest stretches: Repeat five times to each side.

6. Million dollar stretches: Repeat five times.

7. Calf stretches: Repeat five times with each leg.

8. Soleus stretches: Repeat five times with each leg.

9. Double calf stretches: Repeat five times.

10. Double soleus stretches: Repeat five times.

11. Foot sequences: Repeat five times with each foot.

12. Total body stretch: Do at least once a day.

Correcting Coordination

Coordination can be improved with exercise.

Come and learn the best exercises for . . .

CORRECTING COORDINATION

at:

_____

on:

_____

in:

_____

Taught by: _____

LISTEN, LEARN, AND EXERCISE!

CORRECTING COORDINATION

Correcting Coordination

LECTURE/DISCUSSION

Few people stop to think about how their bodies manage to coordinate their movements so that they are smooth and sequenced. Walking, for example, takes a tremendous amount of coordination from the muscles, proprioceptors, and neurons. Every activity involves a certain degree of coordination, however. It was only in 1947 that it was determined which area of the brain stimulates which muscle. Wilder Penfield, a Canadian neurologist, produced a comprehensive map of the cortex, which showed that not all body parts are controlled by the same part of the brain. Furthermore, electrical impulses from many areas of the brain feed into other parts called motor areas. When a movement is executed, all these parts, along with integrated sensory messages, have to be coordinated.

When an illness affects the nervous system, coordination may also be affected. By the same token, certain medications, if not taken as directed or if mixed with other prescribed medications or drugs, such as alcohol, also affect coordination. Parkinson's diesease, Huntington's chorea, and other viral infections are some of the causes of incoordination. Another cause is lack of

practice at certain tasks. Remember what happened the first time you tried to ride a bicycle after years of no practice? You were probably a little wobbly at first, but as you continued to practice, you rode much smoother. Practice and exercise are the solutions to a rusty sense of coordination.

I will give you a handout today with some suggestions on correcting coordination (*Appendix 26-A; read aloud and discuss, if desired*). Now, we are going to do some exercises that are a bit different from others that you have done.

EXERCISES

1. Breathing exercises.
2. Warm-up exercises.
3. Musical body parts. This is a "funny bones" version of musical chairs. Form groups (*by number [e.g., eight], geographic birthplaces [e.g., north, south], etc.*). Begin by finding a partner within your group. I will play music as in musical chairs. When the music stops, I will call out an action that involves connecting to a partner's body part. So, introduce yourself to your partner and touch elbows while the music plays. When the music

stops, find another partner, and listen for other cues. We will do this for about ten body connections.

Other directions for "funny bones" include

(a) Hand to hand
(b) Opposite hand to hand
(c) Knees to knees
(d) Hands to knees
(e) Opposite elbow to opposite shoulder
(f) Back to back
(g) Hip to hip
(h) Heel to ankle
(i) Opposite heel to opposite ankle
(j) High five (arm held high with hand slap) to high five

4. Soap bubbles. I (*or a group leader or volunteer*) will go around to each individual or group and blow bubbles. If you prefer, we can arrange the chairs in a circle. We are going to do this exercise in three parts: (a) individually, while standing; (b) individually, while sitting; and (c) standing or sitting with partners. (*Blowing bubbles correctly takes practice. Do not attempt this exercise without some practice. You are looking for bubbles large enough to minimize spilling of soap.*)

(a) While you are standing, I will blow bubbles way above your heads. As they float down, break the bubbles by clapping your hands together, poking them with your fingers and thumbs, or using your elbows.
(b) While you are seated, break the bubbles by the same methods that you just used, as well as by flutter kicking your feet, pointing your toes, catching them between your knees, or catching them between your feet.
(c) Find a partner, and break the bubbles while I call out the same direc-

tions that we used for funny bones. (*Safety check: Be careful not to blow soap bubbles into participants' eyes or glasses and not to inhale bubbles; wipe up spills immediately, as soap is slippery.*)

5. Eye-foot coordination. (*Lay a strip of red or orange masking tape diagonally across the floor. If you are prohibited from taping anything to the floor, use a roll of lawn chair reweaving material or any other material that lies flat and is secured at both ends. Heavy books at either end may solve the problem.*) Line up for the tight rope walk, also known as the prohibition walk.

(a) We are going to start with an easy task; just walk, taking small steps while straddling the tape.
(b) Walk on the tape sideways with one foot beside the other.
(c) Walk sideways, crossing one foot in front of the other.
(d) Walk sideways, crossing one foot in front of the other, then one foot behind the other.
(e) Walk the tape like a tight rope, with your arms extended, back and forth.

These activities are done best with spotters, and one must always pay attention to the person walking. One can hold races, but not on the first day. These activities have been done in various settings and have proved highly successful for all ambulatory participants, including those with walkers. Modifications are necessary for special cases. Remember that these activities take time; do not rush through them. (*Consider dividing this session into two parts, if necessary.*)

BIBLIOGRAPHY

The Role of the Brain. New York: Time-Life Books, Inc., 1975.

Appendix 26-A

Correcting Coordination Handout

Do's

1. Engage in activities that promote fine motor action of the fingers and hands. Doing certain crafts as hobbies, as well as exercising daily, will stimulate muscle control and coordination.
2. Try different ways of getting your exercise (cross-training). Aquatics, walking, and riding a bicycle place emphasis on specific, but different, muscle groups.
3. Try activities that you have not done in a while. You do not know how "rusty" you are if you do not try.

Don'ts

1. Do not be discouraged if you discover you cannot do a task as well as you could in the past. If you took twenty years to unlearn it, you can spend a few hours a week trying to relearn it.
2. Do not ever say, "I am too old." There is plenty of research to prove that declining abilities are a function of lack of use, not just chronological aging.

Exercises

1. Breathing exercises.
2. Warm-up exercises.
3. Musical body parts.
4. Soap bubbles.
5. Eye-foot coordination.

Understanding Aerobics

What is aerobic exercise? Can people of any age do it? What are the benefits? Is it easy?

Learn the answers to these questions in a class on . . .

UNDERSTANDING AEROBICS

at:

_____

on:

_____

in:

_____

Taught by: _____

LISTEN, LEARN, AND EXERCISE!

UNDERSTANDING AEROBICS

Understanding Aerobics

LECTURE/DISCUSSION

The term *aerobic exercise* refers to rhythmic large muscle activity done at a continuous pace and at a comfortable rate. The goal of aerobic exercise is to raise your heart rate and maintain it. The actual word *aerobic* means ample amounts of oxygen being brought to the muscles.

According to the American College of Sports Medicine, the components of a good aerobic workout are in the acronym FITT: frequency, intensity, time, and type. The frequency of exercise necessary to gain and maintain an aerobic effect is no less than three times per week and no more than five times per week. Anything outside that range may lead to injury. Exercising once or twice a week at various levels of exertion is hazardous, but exercising every day of the week puts a strain on the body. So, use good judgment; start out with three days a week, and slowly increase the frequency until you have reached your goal.

The appropriate intensity can be calculated by measuring heart rate. There are two easy locations for measuring your heart rate: the neck (carotid artery) and the wrist (radial pulse). On the neck, use your finger to palpate the carotid artery, located to the left or right of your windpipe (*demon-*

strate while describing). Do not press too hard, or you will cause your heart rate to fluctuate. Now, count the number of beats per minute in 30-second intervals. Ready, set, go (*pause in silence for 30 seconds*). Stop. Double the number that you just counted, and the result is your heart rate in beats per minute.

Repeat the procedure at the radial pulse (*again, demonstrate while describing*). An easy way to find a radial pulse is to follow the thumb down into the wrist area with the fingertips (fleshy part). The pulse is located in the outer grooves and can be easily found here (*demonstrate*). Repeat the 30-second count, and compare the results.

To determine your target heart rate for exercise, the following formula is used (*Appendix 27-A; use a blackboard or flip chart to explain this process*): Now, I will hand out a worksheet entitled Calculating Your Target Heart Rate. This is the simplest method of getting a ball park estimate of your heart rate. The number "220" is a standard originally developed by a Swedish exercise physiologist. All one has to do is take the number 220 and subtract one's age from it. Once that answer is found, take it and multiply it by 0.65. This number will be the lowest heart rate you want to focus on while doing aerobic work. The number you have just calculated is in beats per minute; that is, the number of heart beats you are effecting per minute.

Now that you all know your safe exercise training heart rate, we need to determine the length of time that you should exercise. Ideally, aerobic exercise should last no less than 15 minutes and no more than 45 minutes; that does not include time for warm-up, cool-down, or any calisthenics. Warm-up exercises are important because they raise your internal body temperature and get you ready for work. This elevation in temperature has a number of physiological benefits, including greater flexibility of tendons and ligaments, increased blood flow to the muscles, and faster nerve impulse transmission. The ultimate purpose of these effects is to reduce the risk of injury. A five- or ten-minute warm-up is particularly important for older adults, because it takes their bodies a little longer to adapt, that is, to elevate the heart rate and to prepare the heart for work. Warm-up exercises may vary. For instance, the warm-up exercises appropriate for a twenty-minute walk differ from those appropriate for cycling, swimming, jogging, or playing tennis. The specificity of exercise is important in preparing your body for the work it is about to face.

It is equally important to cool down after aerobic exercise. Cooling down allows the cardiovascular system to re-establish equilibrium, to return slowly to the resting heart rate. It involves gradually slowing down strenuous movements, progressively reducing the range of motion, stride, pace, or impact. At the end of your allotted aerobic walking time, for example, you should walk slower to decrease your heart rate. You should not stop completely, however. Anytime you stop a vigorous exercise suddenly, you allow blood to pool in your legs. This action can cause you to feel dizzy or even faint, because your blood is not going back up to your heart and head. A failure to cool down adequately can lead to serious physical injury.

Basically, there are three types of exercise: isotonic, isometric, and isokinetic. Aerobic activity, such as walking, swimming, low impact aerobic dance, bicycling, jogging, or racket sports, involves large muscle groups and a full range of motion of the joints. This type of exercise is called isotonic; it is the most effective type of exercise to promote flexibility and cardiovascular endurance. Isometric exercises where there is no range of motion about a joint are the opposite of isotonic exercises and have their place mainly in rehabilitation. Isokinetic exercises require the assistance of a device to take various body parts through a full range of motion, while keeping resistance at a constant level. These are excellent forms of exercise when properly used.

Whatever program you decide to follow, always remember to pace yourself. Start slowly, and gradually build up to a comfortable pace. Do not be discouraged. Remember, it will take you a while to get back into shape. Before we exercise today, I would like to go over some helpful hints (*Appendix 27-B; read aloud and discuss*).

EXERCISES

1. Warm-up routine. (Facilitator: Description of exercises is given in Chapter 4 and in "Lavish Legs.")
   - deep breaths
   - chin tucks
   - shoulder rolls
   - arm stretchers
   - side reaches
   - gentle back arch
   - pelvic tilt
   - leg strengtheners
   - leg spreads
   - ankle bends
   - toe curls
   - ankle circles
   - calf stretches

2. Follow a progression with all forms of exercise. For example, having established your target heart rate, begin an activity for 10 or 15 minutes at a time, and slowly build up. The following are examples of safe programs:

(a) Getting Started Walking Program

(1) Level A. Walk 15 minutes a day at least three times per week. When you are no longer challenged (it becomes too easy), progress to Level B.

(2) Level B. Walk 20 minutes a day at least three times per week. When you are no longer challenged, progress to Level C.

(3) Level C. Walk 20 minutes a day at least four times per week. When you are no longer challenged, progress to Level D.

(4) Level D. Walk 25 minutes a day at least three times per week. When you are no longer challenged, progress to Level E.

(5) Level E. Walk 35 minutes a day at least three times per week. When you are no longer challenged, add another day of walking to your weekly schedule. When that becomes less of a challenge, add five more minutes to your time.

Levels A and B are unlikely to elevate your heart rate to target levels. They are good starter routines for those who have been very sedentary or for those who are overweight, slightly arthritic, or the least flexible, however. Any exercise that you do will be of benefit. As your body adapts itself to your exercise demands, you will learn to increase the number of days you walk while decreasing the time walked. This decrease in time should not be too dramatic— perhaps five to seven minutes at most. Remember that a brisk walk with arms swinging will markedly elevate your heart rate, whereas a lesser pace and natural arm swing will not.

(b) Getting Started Bicycling

(1) Level A. Bicycle on a flat surface for 10 minutes at least three times per week. Do not try to reach your target heart rate; just get used to the bicycle and the feeling for pedaling. When you no longer feel challenged by this routine, go to Level B.

(2) Level B. Bicycle on a flat surface for 20 minutes at least three times per week. Try to keep a steady pace. When you are no longer challenged by this routine, progress to Level C.

(3) Level C. Bicycle for 30 minutes at least three times per week. When you are no longer challenged, go to Level D.

(4) Level D. Bicycle for 30 minutes at least four times per week. When no longer challenged, go to Level E.

(5) Level E. Bicycle for 40 minutes at least three times per week. When no longer challenged, progress to Level F.

(6) Level F. Bicycle for 45 minutes at least three times per week. Progress to Level G when you are no longer challenged by this level.

(7) Level G. Bicycle for 50 minutes at least three times per week. When no longer challenged, progress to Level H.

(8) Level H. Bicycle for any period of time that elevates your heart rate and keeps it at your target level for at least 20 minutes. Be careful not to exhaust your leg muscles. Pedal slowly for two or three minutes, then pedal fast for 2 or 3 minutes. Use

this strategy to build your endurance as you progress throughout this program.

(c) Getting Started Swimming
(1) Level A. Swim with a kickboard for 15 minutes three or four times per week.
(2) Level B. Swim without a kickboard for 15 minutes three or four times per week.
(3) Level C. Using the breast, side, or back stroke or crawl, swim 20 minutes at least three or four times per week.
(4) Level D. Swim for 25 minutes three or four times per week.
(5) Level E. Swim for 30 minutes three or four times per week.

If you decide to use the butterfly stroke occasionally, reduce your time in the water unless you are in good condition. The butterfly stroke is physically more demanding than any of the strokes mentioned in Level C.

REFERENCES

Anderson, Bob. *Stretching*. Bolinas, Calif: Shelter Publications, 1980.

Kuntzleman, Charles, and the editors of Consumer Guide. *The Complete Book of Walking*. New York: Pocket Books, 1979.

Appendix 27-A

Calculating Your Target Heart Rate Handout

My resting heart rate is _____ beats/minute.

My age is _____ years

The formula for target heart rate is
   220 − [My age] = A^*, where A equals age-predicted maximal heart rate.

At 65 percent intensity, A is multiplied by $0.65 = B$ beats/minute, where B equals target heart rate at 65 percent of maximum capacity.

A _____ $\times 0.65 = B$ _____ Beats/minute

A _____ $\times 0.70 = B$ _____ Beats/minute

A _____ $\times 0.75 = B$ _____ Beats/minute

My best option is roughly estimated to be _____ beats/minute.

---

*This is the simplest of formulas, but not the most accurate.

Understanding Aerobics Handout

Hints

1. Wear comfortable clothing, regardless of style. Not all stylish exercise clothes are healthy for you. Any piece of clothing that is too tight is not a good choice.
2. Wear adequate shoes for the activity you are about to perform. Cycling in sandals and no socks is not prudent. Also, walking requires supportive shoes, as does any aerobic dance activity. The most expensive are not always the best, however. Your foot, not your purse, will tell you which shoes fit best.
3. If you take an exercise class from a community facility or health club, find out about the qualifications of the instructor. Most good instructors are certified. The International Dance-Exercise Association, for example, has a rigorous, comprehensive written examination for its instructors.
4. If you are unmotivated, join a group whose members are about your age or are in the same physical condition.

5. If you are handicapped in any way, consider buying an exercise video that addresses your restrictions.
6. If you join an exercise class and can-not keep up with the instructor, do the routine at your own pace. Your personal safety comes before everything else.

Do's

1. Warm up every time that you exercise.
2. Take your heart rate after warming up to see if you are approaching your target heart rate.
3. Take your heart rate within ten seconds immediately after stopping the aerobic portion of your workout. This is an important reading of your cardiovascular level of fitness.
4. Cool down every time that you exercise.
5. Take your heart rate within ten seconds of your cool-down period. If your heart rate is still too high (not within five beats of your

resting heart rate), continue to cool down.

Don'ts

1. Do not exercise aerobically fewer than three times per week. You will be gaining little benefit.

2. Do not exercise at erratic times of the week. Plan a schedule, and stick to it.

3. Do not perform aerobic activities before bedtime. You will be refreshed, not tired, and will have trouble sleeping.

All about Alzheimer's Disease

Do you wonder about memory loss? or Do you wonder how to stay mentally stimulated?

Learn the answers to these questions in a class . . .

ALL ABOUT ALZHEIMER'S DISEASE

at:

_____

on:

_____

in:

_____

Taught by: _____

LISTEN, LEARN, AND EXERCISE!

ALL ABOUT ALZHEIMER'S DISEASE

All about Alzheimer's Disease

LECTURE/DISCUSSION

Older people often worry about the loss of their mental faculties. Although normal aging does not disturb them, they fear that an intellectual or memory impairment will debilitate them. Those who have a family member who has suffered a stroke or is a victim of Alzheimer's disease know all too well how frustrating it can be for that family member to perform the activities of daily living and other tasks. The sadness that these diseases bring upon the family can be long-lasting and exhausting.

It has been estimated that, of the 7 to 9 percent of adults over the age of 65 who have some type of dementia, the majority (four million) have Alzheimer's disease, a progressive, degenerative disease that attacks the brain, slowly incapacitating its victim. Alzheimer's is democratic with respect to education, race, socioeconomic level, and sex; there are more women with Alzheimer's simply because women live longer. It also appears to run in families.

Multi-infarct dementia is a cognitive impairment caused by a series of small strokes. Its cause is known (e.g., high blood pressure, advanced arteriosclerosis or atherosclerosis, or possibly alcohol abuse), and it can be treated with medica-tion and rehabilitation, if the stroke is not too severe. In contrast, the cause of Alzheimer's is unknown, and the prognosis for rehabilitation is poor.

The signs of Alzheimer's include changes in three or more of the following five areas:

1. Memory of a rote skill, particularly if it is a job-related skill, hobby, or sport.
2. Judgment, that is, the inability to make a good, quick, or clear judgment.
3. Intellectual functioning. A simple matter of making change from a dollar bill or not being able to make sense of a phrase or proverb commonly heard may signal a problem.
4. Orientation. A victim of Alzheimer's may leave the house to go for a walk and become disoriented in a neighborhood where he or she has lived for 20 years. The person may also be disoriented as to people, places, and time.
5. Mood swings and radical changes in personality.

Because the side effects of many medications may include behavioral changes in any or all of these areas, always seek a professional diagnosis from a geriatrician, neurologist, or geriatric psychologist.

Before you leave today, I will give you a handout with hints on how to stay alert (*Appendix 28-A; read aloud and discuss, if desired*).

EXERCISE ROUTINES FOR VICTIMS OF DEMENTIA

Structure is very important to the person with Alzheimer's. A consistent exercise routine done at the same time every day or every other day renders positive results. Exercising regularly not only improves the physical condition of a person with Alzheimer's, but also causes fatigue, which in turn may help the person sleep better.

Instructions given to the exerciser should be as brief and direct as possible. Give one directive at a time, then slowly continue. If the individual cannot follow even the briefest direction, simply say "Do what I do." The exerciser is likely to mimic you. Do not be too concerned with form unless the exercises are for rehabilitative purposes. For example, if you are modeling for the exerciser to do large arm circles clockwise, and the exerciser does small arm circles in a clockwise direction, be patient. It is the movement that you are after, not comprehension and interpretation of direction.

Use music for the exercise routines. Music is soothing, energizing, motivating, and nostalgic. Magic happens with "just the right song." If the exerciser wants to dance in the middle of a warm up, do not become discouraged. For reasons not quite yet understood, dancing is one skill that does not diminish in individuals with Alzheimer's, despite severe declines in coordination or ambulation. Dancing can be an excellent form of exercise and an opportunity for touching and tenderness.

If the individual has very short attention or concentration abilities, keep the exercise routine down to a minimum. In fact, you may want to intersperse exercise throughout the week, for short durations (five to ten minutes). If whatever activity you are doing at home is not perceived as fun by the exerciser, do not force the issue. Look for other ways to promote cardiovascular health, such as walking briskly in malls (window shopping), playing catch with a ball, playing horseshoes or indoor bowling (all materials should be plastic), or kneading clay to make things. This last activity is also good for the caregiver who has arthritic hands.

If you are exercising with someone who is in the "early" stages of Alzheimer's, you will be able to follow a comprehensive exercise routine that includes warm-up (five minutes), flexibility exercises (ten minutes), aerobic activity (fifteen minutes), and cool-down (more flexibility exercises for ten minutes).

In summary, the following rules apply to exercise programs for persons with dementia:

1. The exercise activity should take place in a calm environment.
2. Structure and routine should prevail over spontaneity and surprise.
3. Directions should be brief, to the point, and slowly given.
4. Music may be used as a stimulant and a pacifier.
5. Fun should be a strong goal of the exercise session.
6. Patience, kindness of tone and attitude, and sources of affection should be constant.

EXERCISES

Facilitator: use warm-up routine (Chapter 4), aerobics, flexibility, relaxation, and breathing handouts as sample routines.

Appendix 28-A

All about Alzheimer's Disease Handout

Do's

1. Remain mentally active. Nourish the brain with intellectual stimulation, such as crossword puzzles, reading, wordfinder and jigsaw puzzles, and computer games that require intellectual decisions.
2. Remain physically active. A healthy body means adequate circulation to all areas of the body, especially the brain. Fitness is achievable at any age.
3. Get plenty of quality sleep. Sleep patterns change with age, but getting adequate sleep and knowing when to rest are always important.
4. Stay emotionally close to good friends if family members are not geographically close to you. A close friend in whom to confide and with whom to be playful is very important to mental health.
5. Eat plenty of grains, legumes, fruits, and vegetables. Keep red meats and foods high in fat to a minimum. Poultry, turkey, and fish are better choices.
6. If you find that you cannot "shake off" the blues, consider speaking to a professional who will help you. Although not synonymous with depression, "the blues" can lead to protracted periods of bad feelings.
7. Keep a positive attitude. It is never too late to improve attitude.

Don'ts

1. Do not worry about things over which you have no control. Wondering "what if" is a dangerous game. Live each day to its fullest, not in fear of what might be.
2. Do not take anyone else's medication. What may be good for a friend's symptoms may be disastrous for you.
3. Do not ignore signs of depression. Talk to friends or seek professional help, including the help of your clergy.

Exercises

1. Daily stretches and warm-ups

   - Deep breaths
   - Chin tucks
   - Shoulder rolls
   - Arm stretchers
   - Side reaches
   - Gentle back arch
   - Pelvic tilt
   - Leg strengtheners
   - Leg spreads
   - Ankle bends
   - Toe curls
   - Ankle circles

2. Daily walks. Escort the individual with dementia as you walk around your neighborhood, up and down your apartment corridors, or along a local school track. Use this opportunity to dis-cover pleasant or amusing sights. If the individual becomes alarmed due to disorientation, gently help the individual to walk back toward "home."

3. Dancing. Dancing can be done within the confines of your own home. It is not unlikely that this form of exercise will become routine pleasure for both partners. Try to incorporate dances that meet the goal of maintaining range of motion and subtle stretching. The "hokey pokey" is a good example.

4. Relaxation. Practicing deep breathing before the person goes to bed may be effective in relaxing the individual initially. Also, it can be used as a routine cue to prepare the individual for bed. As the disease progresses, however, the idea of cuing becomes less effective.

Achieving Perfect Body Weight

What is the correct body weight for you? Can exercise help you to control your weight?

Learn about . . .

ACHIEVING PERFECT BODY WEIGHT

at:

_____

on:

_____

in:

_____

Taught by: _____

LISTEN, LEARN, AND EXERCISE!

ACHIEVING PERFECT BODY WEIGHT

Achieving Perfect Body Weight

LECTURE/DISCUSSION

One thing we all have in common is a concern about our weight. Some people need to gain weight, while others need to lose it. The latter is the much larger group, by far. We no longer consider weight only in terms of actual weight, however. Rather, we speak of fat weight, that is, the percentage of body fat. If you are 20 percent over your ideal weight, the odds are good that your body fat is higher than it should be.

The concept of weight management usually brings to mind the word *diet*. A more constructive phrase would be *life style*, meaning that, if you eat in a healthy way all your life, the odds are good that you will maintain a healthy weight. Of course, not only what we eat, but also how much we eat is what weight management is really all about.

Dietary Guidelines

It has been known for years that there are four food groups: (1) milk, (2) meat, (3) fruits and vegetables, and (4) grains and cereals. Over the years, we have learned that excessive amounts of any one food are harmful, that a diet high in fat is

deadly, that excessive consumption of salt and refined sugars is harmful, that supplementing our daily food intake with excessive amounts of minerals and vitamins can wreak havoc with the body's electrolytes or negatively react with prescribed medications; that high consumption of fiber is cancer preventive, and that alcohol consumption should be limited. These facts have remained constant. The dietary recommendations made by the American Heart Association have changed over these years, however. It is now known that the bulk of our food intake, 58 percent, should come from complex carbohydrates and naturally occurring sugars. Of that 58 percent, only 10 percent should come from refined sugars, such as those used in cakes and cookies, while 48 percent should come from complex carbohydrates, such as fruits and vegetables. Also, 30 percent of our daily intake should come from fats, and only 12 percent should come from proteins.

Carbohydrates

A simple carbohydrate is mostly composed of refined sugars, such as those found in doughnuts, cakes, cookies, and assorted pastries. The primary ingredient in these foods is sugar. By comparison, complex carbohydrates contain fiber and natural sugars from fruits and vegetables.

Fiber exists in two forms: insoluble and soluble. Insoluble fiber in adequate amounts reduces constipation and keeps the bowels working smoothly. Soluble fiber binds with cholesterol (i.e., low-density lipoprotein) in the body and helps to eliminate it. Insoluble fiber is found in wheat, bran, and greens. Foods high in soluble fiber are potatoes, peas, bananas, pears, chick peas, pinto and lima beans, and oats. Nuts, such as almonds, pecans, and walnuts, are also high in fiber; however, they are also high in fat, so they should be eaten sparingly. It is recommended that you have one or two servings of foods high in dietary fiber at each meal.

Fats

There are three types of fats: saturated fats, monosaturated fats, and polyunsaturated fats. Saturated fats contribute to elevations in the cholesterol level, especially the low-density lipoprotein level. For this reason, eating foods high in saturated fats increases the risk of heart attack, stroke, and high blood pressure. The two other kinds of fats, monosaturated and polyunsaturated, are far less harmful to the body.

Saturated fats are found primarily in red meats, such as steak, sausage, strip bacon, and luncheon meats. They are also contained in dairy products, such as butter, whole milk, hard cheeses, ice cream, and they are hidden in processed or packaged foods that contain certain oils, such as coconut, cottonseed, or palm oils, or lard. Foods high in fats are usually high in calories as well. Choosing fewer fatty foods and more low-fat foods will accomplish two important objectives; it will reduce the number of calories ingested and decrease the risk of heart disease and obesity.

Protein

Most of the protein in our diet comes from meat, poultry, game, and fish. Other sources are nuts and cheeses. The body does not require large amounts of protein, as reflected in the daily requirement of only 12 percent. The amount of fat within that 12 percent of protein can be controlled by selecting chicken and fish over red meats and organ meats, which are highest in cholesterol, and by trimming the fat off foods before they are cooked, which includes removing the skin from chicken. Cooking habits are also important here. For example, baking, broiling, poaching, stewing, and barbecuing without the skin are healthier ways to cook than are pan frying, deep frying, blackening (as in Creole cooking), or barbecuing until food is charred.

Calorie Counting

Whether they come from ice cream or a tossed salad, 100 calories are 100 calories. The content of the calories is not always equal, however. The 100 calories of ice cream are high in saturated fat, whereas the 100 calories of a tossed salad are high in fiber and loaded with vitamins and minerals.

Not all foods contain the same number of calories per unit. For example, fats contain 9 calories per gram, proteins and carbohydrates contain 4 calories per gram, and alcohol contains 7 calories per gram. Therefore, the first rule of weight management is to know the quality of foods. This is an ongoing learning process that requires reading labels, studying the contents of a package, and referring to other materials that list the nutritive values of various foods.

The next rule is to know your daily caloric expenditure. A person with a sedentary life style does not need as many calories to stay healthy as does someone who exercises regularly. There are several ways to calculate this number. A crude method is to use a paper-and-pencil formula; a more sophisticated method involves a battery of tests with scientific equipment to calculate your metabolic rate. No matter what your situation, active or passive, you should never eat less than 1,200 calories per day. The body requires nutrients just as a car requires gasoline. If the tank is running low, the car eventually slows down and stops. If a person eats too little food, the body slows down the rate at which calories are burned. Sometimes, this is the explanation of the plateau effect, where, no matter what little food is eaten, the body does not lose weight.

Another rule for weight loss is exercise, exercise, exercise. Walk, swim, ride a bike, swing your arms, take the stairs, park farther from the door of a store and walk farther to shop, but do it. There is no way a weight loss program can be effective without exercise. Losing weight and keeping it off requires exercising and watching food intake. Every movement counts, no matter how small. Remember, walking is still one of the best exercises!

If you are unable to move around as much as you would like, ask a registered dietitian to help you with a plan of action that takes into consideration your inability to exercise. Your personal physician may have a recommendation regarding the number of calories that you should be consuming.

The most comforting rule is to allow yourself all kinds of foods in small quantities; never deny yourself a food for the wrong reason. It is not necessary to refuse all desserts or sauces on foods for fear of gaining weight. Learn to plan ahead and reward yourself. For example, if you eat only low-fat foods, but are out to dinner or visiting a friend, it is all right to have a small amount of a food item that you would not otherwise make or buy for yourself. Choosing wisely, learning to trade one food for another, and understanding what makes the body healthy is what counts.

A long-standing, but often forgotten, rule is to drink plenty of water. Water helps to cleanse the body, to move digested food through the body, and to keep the skin from drying out. Water also fills you up when you are not really hungry; satisfying

a need to ingest while helping the digestion and elimination process as well.

A more recent rule of weight management is to be consistent with eating patterns. Many people try different diets on and off for months or years. This is known as yo-yo dieting. The body is pretty smart. If it does not get enough calories, it starts to slow down the rate at which it burns these fewer calories. It generally returns to its normal metabolism when the number of calories increases. When this pattern happens regularly, however, the yo-yo effect eventually leads the body to burn calories slower overall.

There is a great deal of controversy over which is more effective, eating several small meals during the day or eating three square meals a day. Regardless of which method you use, eat breakfast. Study after study has shown that people who skip breakfast eat more at later times of the day when their activity level has decreased and they are less likely to burn the calories that they have consumed.

People who are overweight weigh more than they should for someone of their sex, height, and frame size. A crude, but acceptable, measure of frame size is to place your thumb and middle (longest) finger around the wrist of your nonpreferred hand. For example, if you are right-handed, place your right thumb and middle finger around your left wrist. If your thumb and middle finger overlap by at least ¼ inch or more, you have a small frame. If your finger and thumb touch, you have a medium frame. If they do not touch, you have a large frame.

Scales do not know the difference, however, between fat pounds and muscle pounds. Muscle weighs more than fat. So, if you are exercising to become firm and in better shape, it may sometimes appear that you have gained weight. Try to weigh yourself at the same time of day about twice a week to see how you are doing. Weighing in every day is not recommended. Before you leave today, I will give you a handout with some do's and don'ts for weight management (*Appendix 29-A; read aloud and discuss, if desired*).

NUTRITION EDUCATION ACTIVITIES

It is recommended that the class on nutrition be conducted in a minimum of two segments. The first segment should focus on re-educating the class participants in the fundamentals of good eating habits. In order to enhance this class, it is recommended that the training package *Culinary Hearts Kitchen* be purchased from your local branch of the American Heart Association for a nominal fee ($65 at this writing). This kit contains excellent slides and a training manual. Also, the association has free pamphlets available for distribution.

Another excellent resource is the American Dairy Association. Once again, educational materials may be purchased. Items such as food cutouts in their ideal portion sizes, colorful one-page handouts representing the four basic food groups, and training programs are also available.

The second segment should focus on establishing a reasonable caloric intake for each class participant. Once the participants have a goal to reach, discussions of the need for exercise, weight management techniques, and the possibility of joining a group for support and accountability may be added. There are several weight loss programs from which to choose. Investigate the ones in your area before making recommendations.

An ideal reference is *Jane Brody's Nutrition Book*, Chapter 16, "Why Diets Don't Work." Another good resource is *Setting Your Weight*, one of a series from Time-Life's Fitness, Health, and Nutrition Series. You may also want to visit support groups, such as Overeaters Anonymous, a group that deals with compulsive eating behavior. It is also helpful to go to the library and read back issues of the *Tuft's University Nutrition Newsletter*. It is invaluable in content and will give you excellent material for extra handouts.

BIBLIOGRAPHY

American Heart Association. *The American Heart Association Cookbook.* New York: Ballantine Books, 1984.

Brody, Jane. *Jane Brody's Nutrition Book.* New York: Bantam Books, Inc., 1987.

Setting Your Weight. Alexandria, Va.: Time-Life Books, Inc., 1987.

Appendix 29-A

Achieving Perfect Body Weight Handout

Do's

1. Know your ideal weight.
2. Learn about the difference between cholesterol-containing foods and saturated fat–containing foods. Remember that only animal products contain cholesterol. When a food item is marked "no cholesterol," it does not necessarily mean "no fat."
3. Think about eating all foods in moderation. Remember that not all calories are created equal.
4. Shop wisely. Read labels. Buy fresh vegetables and fruits whenever possible.
5. Ask the supermarket manager if there are guided tours of the store by registered dietitians. Often, groups of interested parties are taken on a tour of the grocery store in conjunction with the American Heart Association's *Culinary Heart's Kitchen* program, as well as part of other educational programs sponsored by a local health maintenance organization or hospital.

Don'ts

1. Do not weigh yourself every day. Body fluids fluctuate, and it takes a few days to show changes in weight loss or gain.
2. Do not take weight loss for granted. If you have been experiencing rapid weight loss, combined with excessive thirst and frequent urination, you may have adult-onset diabetes. Consult your doctor immediately.
3. Do not play with liquid or powdered diets or mineral and herbal supplements, especially if you are on medication. Think of your body as a test tube. Every individual will react differently to something extra that enters the body.
4. Do not use laxatives or enemas as weight regulators. Eat foods rich in fiber (complex carbohydrates) daily, and exercise. These two actions combined should help prevent constipation.
5. Do not try to lose weight by yourself if you are not motivated or have a difficult time changing bad habits. Rely on friends who know you well for support. Remember that the most important person is you, however.

Exercising Facial Muscles

Facelifts cost thousands of dollars.

Instead of having a facelift, come and learn about . . .

EXERCISING FACIAL MUSCLES

at:

_____

on:

_____

in:

_____

Taught by: _____

LISTEN, LEARN, AND EXERCISE!

EXERCISING FACIAL MUSCLES

Exercising Facial Muscles

LECTURE/DISCUSSION

We will not actually be giving you a face-lift today, but we will be teaching you exercises to strengthen and tone your facial muscles. The face actually has quite a few muscles (*hold up a picture of the face with all the different muscles outlined*). All the muscles in the body tend to atrophy as we get older, more because of disuse than because of actual aging. This is also true of the muscles in the face.

There are many muscles all over the face and around the hairline that can be strengthened with activities. Close your eyes as tight as you can, and relax. You just strengthened one of the muscles around your eyes. Puff your lips as if you are kissing. That is another example. Obviously, you will not look like you have had a face-lift, but you may feel a little relief from tension if you learn to tighten and relax the muscles around your face and neck area. You may also have fewer muscle spasms and headaches. I will give you a handout today to help you remember how to exercise your facial muscles (*Appendix 30-A; read aloud and discuss, if desired*).

EXERCISES

1. Chawing. Chaw, not chew, bubble gum for five minutes daily.
2. Ah-h-h-ing. Say "ah-h-h," prolonging the sound for five seconds. Repeat five times (Figure 30-1).
3. Grin and pucker. Grin, then pucker your lips (Figure 30-2). Repeat five times.
4. Cheek blow and suck. Blow out, then suck in your cheek. Repeat five times.
5. Tongue touches. Pretend your tongue is cleaning food from between your cheek and teeth. Repeat five times.
6. Exaggerator. Speak or read with exaggerated mouth movements for short intervals several times daily. Repeat five times.
7. Making faces. Make faces at yourself in a mirror (Figure 30-3). Repeat five times.
8. Shoulder circles. Bring shoulders around in big circles, three times clockwise and three times counterclockwise.

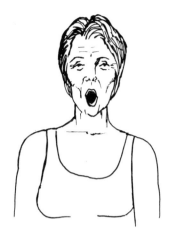

Figure 30-1 Vowel Sounds "Ah"

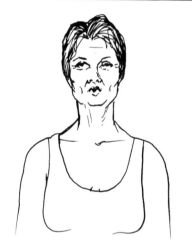

Figure 30-2 Pucker

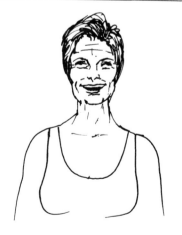

Figure 30-3 Making Faces

9. Chin tucks. Stand as erect as you can, with your neck drawn back and your chin tucked in, not up. Do not tilt your chin. Pull your neck back in line with your spine, keeping your chin horizontal. Hold this position for ten seconds. Relax. Breathe. Repeat three times.

10. Eye openers. Open your eyes to the maximum extent possible for a slow count of six. It is additionally helpful while you are holding them open to look to the right, to the left, above, and below. Repeat three times.

11. Nose wrinklers. Contract the muscles on either side of the nose as you do in sneezing, wrinkling the skin over the nose upward as hard as you can. Repeat three times.

12. Nose openers. Dilate the nostrils. Flare them out. Repeat three times.

13. Mouth movers. Pull first the right and then the left corner of the mouth up and out. Hold each position six seconds. Repeat three times.

14. Frowners. Pull first the right and then the left corner of the mouth down and out (Figure 30-4). Hold each position. Repeat three times.

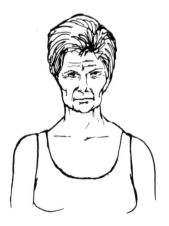

Figure 30-4 Frowner

15. Lower lipping. Pull the lower lip down as vigorously as possible, keeping it flat. Do not evert (turn outward) the lower lip. Repeat three times.
16. Kissing. Make a movement of the lips as if you were kissing or whistling, but do it extremely vigorously. Repeat three times.
17. Big mouths. Open your mouth as wide as you possibly can in all directions, and hold. Repeat three times.

Exercising Facial Muscles Handout

Do's

1. Exercise your facial muscles as often as possible without causing headaches or increased pain.
2. Try to do the exercises in a relatively relaxed manner; do not tighten your facial muscles so severely that it hurts you.
3. Relax your facial muscles as much as you actively contract them.
4. Use expressions with your facial muscles as often as possible.
5. Relax your muscles when you are not actively tightening them.

Don'ts

1. Do not keep the muscles in your face tense all the time.
2. Do not exercise your facial muscles constantly.

Exercises

1. Chawing: Do five minutes daily.
2. Ah-h-h-ing: Repeat five times.
3. Grin and pucker: Repeat five times.
4. Cheek blow and suck: Repeat five times.
5. Tongue touches: Repeat five times.
6. Exaggerator: Repeat five times.
7. Making faces: Repeat five times.
8. Shoulder shrugs: Repeat three times clockwise and three times counterclockwise.
9. Chin tucks. Repeat three times.
10. Eye openers: Repeat three times.
11. Nose wrinklers: Repeat three times.
12. Nose openers: Repeat three times.
13. Mouth movers: Repeat three times.
14. Frowners: Repeat three times.
15. Lower lipping: Repeat three times.
16. Kissing: Repeat three times.
17. Big mouths: Repeat three times.

Hidden Exercises

"I don't have time to exercise." For those of you who don't have time to exercise, come join us in our class on . . .

HIDDEN EXERCISES

at:

_____

on:

_____

in:

_____

Taught by: _____

LISTEN, LEARN, AND EXERCISE!

HIDDEN EXERCISES

Hidden Exercises

LECTURE/DISCUSSION

The biggest problem with sitting too much is that some muscles become tight, while others grow weak. If, for example, you sit at a desk all the time, your hip flexors, which are right where the hip bends, will tighten with the hip at a right angle. While those muscles get stronger and tighter, the hip muscles in the behind (*point to your gluteals*) will get weaker because they are overstretched in that position. In addition, the pectoral muscles (*indicate where the pectoral muscles are*) across your chest can get very tight, while the muscles along your back (*indicate where these muscles are*) can get very weak. Therefore, it is necessary to do exercises to stretch out those muscles and to strengthen the other muscles.

The exercises that we are going to do today can be done while sitting around the television or at a desk. They are especially good, if you sit too much. Before you leave today, I will give you a handout with helpful hints to remember if you must sit at a desk or in a chair for long periods of time (*Appendix 31-A; read aloud and discuss, if desired*).

EXERCISES

1. Hip circles. Stand in front of a mirror, and try to make a circle with your hips without moving your shoulders. Repeat ten times.
2. Chin tucks. Stand erect with your neck drawn back and your chin tucked in. Do not tilt your chin. Pull your neck back in line with your spine, keeping your chin horizontal. Hold for ten seconds. Repeat three times.
3. Back and upper body extensions. Place your hands in the small of your back, and gently arch backward. Repeat three times.
4. Wrist flexions. Gently apply force with the left palm to stretch the right wrist toward the underside of the right forearm. Hold for three to five seconds, and then repeat with other side. Repeat five times with each wrist.
5. Wrist hyperextensions. Gently apply force with the left hand to bend the right hand backward. Hold for three to five seconds. Relax. Repeat five times.

6. Front and lateral flexions. (Head tilts.) Slowly bend your head to the left, then to the right, then forward. Relax. Repeat seven times.

7. Hugs. Stand erect, bring your arms across your chest, trying to touch as far around the back as possible. Hold for ten seconds, and relax. Repeat three to five times.

8. Wall stretchers. Face a wall about three feet away, and lean into the wall with arms extended. Slowly bend your left leg toward the wall until you feel a stretch in your right leg. Keep your feet flat on the floor at all times. Hold the position for three to five seconds. Relax; repeat with the other leg. Repeat each two times.

9. Fencer's lunges. With your feet twice your shoulders' width apart and your right foot pointing out to the side, bend your right knee while keeping your left leg straight. You should feel a slight pulling sensation in your inner thigh. Hold the position three to five seconds. Relax; then repeat with the other leg. Repeat each five times.

10. Look behinds. Stand erect, feet shoulder width apart, arms extended to the side with the palms facing up. Twist to the right at the waist, and look as far behind you as possible. Hold for three to five seconds. Relax; then repeat to the left side. Repeat each three times.

11. Side stretches. Extend your left hand straight overhead, and place your right hand on your hip. Lean as far as comfortable to the right. Come back to the starting position, relax, and repeat with the opposite hand. Hold each stretch seven to ten seconds. Repeat three to five times each.

12. Seated stretches. Sit in a chair, feet flat on the floor, knees no more than 12 inches apart, hands at sides. Bend over as far as comfortable, and reach toward or touch the floor. Hold position for three to five seconds. Return to starting position; relax. Repeat three to five times.

13. Shoulder shrugs. Bring your shoulders up to your ears. Relax. Repeat five times.

Appendix 31-A

Hidden Exercises Handout

Hints

1. Exercise as often as possible.
2. Try to move around, changing chairs and positions, so that your various muscles do not become tight.

Do's

1. Get up as often as possible.
2. Move your hips around.
3. Do exercises every hour.
4. If you are watching television, get up and stand for every commercial.

Don'ts

1. Do not sit in one position too long.
2. Do not bend forward over a desk for longer than one-half hour.
3. Do not accept tightness in your hip muscles as normal aging.

Exercises

1. Hip circles: Do this ten times.
2. Chin tucks: Hold for ten seconds, and repeat three times.
3. Back and upper body extensions: Repeat three times.
4. Wrist flexions: Repeat five times with each wrist.
5. Wrist hyperextensions: Repeat five times.
6. Front and lateral flexions: Repeat seven times.
7. Hugs: Repeat three to five times.
8. Wall stretches: Repeat two times.
9. Fencer's lunges: Repeat five times.
10. Look behinds: Repeat three times.
11. Side stretches: Repeat three to five times.
12. Seated stretches: Repeat three to five times.
13. Shoulder shrugs: Repeat five times.

Part III

Special Considerations, Program Evaluation, and Follow-Up

32

Special Considerations

In any class setting, special considerations may arise. Among the most common are situations in which the class leader must determine how to deal with wheelchair-bound participants, how to incorporate paraplegics or amputees into activity sessions, how to conduct class activities when participants do not understand English, how to deal with participants who demand too much attention or are disruptive, and how to manage participants with dementia.

WHEELCHAIR-BOUND PARTICIPANTS

There is nothing wheelchair-bound participants cannot do unless they are restricted by a physical condition, such as an inability to move certain body parts. No special directions are necessary for these participants other than to make certain that their wheelchair brakes are not on when they are moving from one location to the next. Also, the leader should feel comfortable when handling a wheelchair and should be aware of certain important safety considerations.

1. Always make sure the brakes are OK when doing exercises.

2. If the individual would like to stand for an activity, make certain the brakes are on and the foot rests are out of the way.

3. Always keep a wheelchair-bound individual's feet from dragging on the floor when the wheelchair is positioned for exercises or group activity. Have the individual use the foot rests.

4. If the participant is a double leg amputee, add a weight to the front of the chair at the leg rest or front of the seat. This will prevent tipping.

5. Make sure the participant has adequate balance, so that reaching movements do not cause him or her to fall out of the chair. Use a seat belt when one is available.

6. When wheeling the individual, do not stop suddenly, lurching the individual forward. The person in the chair trusts you; do not jeopardize that.

7. When wheeling into a room, it is proper to wheel person-forward. When wheeling into an elevator, however, wheel in backward. You can control the chair better that way.

8. When wheeling down an incline or over a curb, also wheel backward to prevent the person from spilling out of the chair. It takes practice to wheel

off a curb that is not wheelchair-accessible. You must tilt the chair toward you by stepping on the low bar facing you when the chair is turned backward. Use the handles to press out and down. Do not exceed an angle of 35 degrees when tilting. Use your body to support the weight of the chair.

9. When speaking to the individual in a chair, meet the person at eye level. This will require you to bend at the knees and crouch. Placing yourself at the side of the chair is most comfortable.

PARAPLEGIC AND AMPUTEE PARTICIPANTS

Occasionally, someone without the use of half his or her body joins an activity class. Paraplegics who come to such classes know their limitations. They often adapt to the situation and enjoy the camaraderie. Unless such an individual appears to be uncomfortable, it is not necessary to approach him or her. If, however, you are doing a leg exercise or a class activity that entails the use of the lower limbs, ask the individual to assist you with class-related activities. Participation at any level is the goal.

Regardless of the site of amputation, amputees themselves will take on the responsibility of adapting to an exercise class. Watch for signs of overuse or overexertion, however. Experience has shown that an individual who cannot follow an exercise or activity because a specific body part is missing may overcompensate.

PARTICIPANTS WHO DO NOT SPEAK ENGLISH

As do hearing-impaired older adults, participants in an exercise class who do not speak English need visual cues, an unobstructed view, voice inflections, and body language to replace the spoken word. If the class is didactic in nature, do not ignore these individuals; make eye contact and include them when passing out handouts. Often, handouts are later interpreted by friends or family members. Whatever the case, always greet these participants by saying "Hello" and shaking hands or touching their hands in a friendly and reassuring manner.

DISRUPTIVE PARTICIPANTS

An old trick is to ignore a disruptive individual as much as possible during a session. That includes not making eye contact with the individual and ignoring constant questions that interrupt the session. Assuming that the individual is not cognitively or psychologically impaired, ask to speak to the individual after a particularly difficult session and tell him or her that you will be happy to answer any questions after the session is over. You may also ask the individual to help you with certain tasks, such as attendance records, handing out and collecting name tags, helping to lead certain activities, or being the safety watchdog. Disruptive behaviors are often demands for attention. There are ways to settle matters without hurting anyone's feelings.

PARTICIPANTS WITH SIGNS OF DEMENTIA

One of the most difficult situations arises when a participant shows signs of dementia, although the condition has not been diagnosed. Speak to the person who directs the facility or the immediate health professional in charge of the unit. Discuss what you are observing, particularly changes over time or peculiar behaviors. It may be necessary to contact the individual's immediate family.

BIBLIOGRAPHY

Christensen, Alice, and David Rankin. *Easy Does It Yoga for Older People*. New York: Harper & Row, 1975.

Hurley, Olga. *Safe Therapeutic Exercise for the Frail Elderly: An Introduction*. Boston: 1986.

33

Program Evaluation and Follow-Up

The overall goal of a health promotion program is to reduce the risk of disease by changing personal health-related behavior. Although noble in its long-term objectives, such a program is not easy to measure. In evaluating your program, you must determine whether you are evaluating the efficacy of your intervention based on qualitative measures (i.e., increased flexibility, lowered resting heart rate) or the effects of socialization, increases in social support systems, or secondary caregiving to name a few.

Health promotion efforts in working with the older adult involves modifying their behavior. Such a task is difficult with adults at any age, but older adults have a track record of noncompliance with treatment regimens. Furthermore, although a life style behavior may be changeable, reducing the overall risk may not be possible. Presently, there is a paucity of research in this specific area, despite the increase in epidemiological studies. There is another question related to the effect of risk reduction, particularly if the risk factors are a result of a pre-existing condition. If a risk factor has existed for an extended period of time, what are the odds that it will disappear or be totally alleviated?

At the present time, there is a lack of direction for health promotion efforts with the older populations. Although research findings support the prevention of disease and disability among the elderly through exercise programs, there are no unconditional guarantees for interventions in this age group. This fact should not be discouraging. Of all the health promotion interventions given (e.g., cholesterol control, smoking cessation, and stress or weight management), exercise has been proved effective for preventive, interventive, and postventive measures; however, efficacy and compliance remain key issues at all ages. Many interventions will be measured in psychosocial parameters. If no other measure is reliable or applicable and if that meets your original objective, there is nothing wrong with it.

SIMPLE EVALUATION FOR FUTURE PROGRAM DEVELOPMENT

As the program leader, you will want to keep data on demographic variables as well as class attendance for attrition rates. You may discover trends that will help you to

Table 33-1 Checklist Used To Evaluate Exercise or Activity Programs

Criteria	Poor (1)	Fair (2)	Good (3)	Very Good (4)	Excellent (5)
1. Does the program contain a diversity of activities to meet the needs and interests of all its participants?	____	____	____	____	____
2. Does the program contain an adequate balance of physical, psychosocial, intellectual, and spiritual activities?	____	____	____	____	____
3. Are the activities compatible with the philosophy and objectives of the organization?	____	____	____	____	____
4. Do the activities offered meet the needs of both sexes and of varied socioeconomic groups?	____	____	____	____	____
5. Does the program contain an appropriate balance of individual and group activities?	____	____	____	____	____
6. Does the program reflect considerable interest, enthusiasm, and satisfaction by the participants?	____	____	____	____	____
7. Does the program include volunteers and other senior adult leaders with unique talents in the conduct of activities?	____	____	____	____	____
8. Is the program directed by professionally qualified leadership compatible with the job requirements?	____	____	____	____	____
9. Are the activities scheduled at appropriate times during the day and evening hours?	____	____	____	____	____
10. Does the program offer activities whereby participants have an opportunity to learn new intellectual and motor skills?	____	____	____	____	____
11. Is the activity area large enough and properly equipped for the safe conduct of various social and recreational activities?	____	____	____	____	____
12. Does the facility contain a gymnasium or fitness activity area, as well as ready access to a natatorium?	____	____	____	____	____
13. Are all potential safety hazards, including lighting, furniture arrangements, floor composition, stairs, and passageways, reduced to a minimum to allow easy access to and from one point to another in the facility?	____	____	____	____	____
14. Are procedures for emergency situations that may arise clearly defined and known by the staff and participants?	____	____	____	____	____
15. Does the facility contain adequate toilet accommodations that can be quickly reached and easily used?	____	____	____	____	____
16. Is the equipment used in good working order?	____	____	____	____	____
17. Does the program of activities reflect evidence of careful planning?	____	____	____	____	____
18. Does the program of activities reflect good communications among staff members?	____	____	____	____	____
19. Are the facility and program adequately funded?	____	____	____	____	____
20. Is the facility attractive and amenable to a relaxing ambience?	____	____	____	____	____

Source: Reprinted from *Fitness and Aging* by John Piscopo, pp. 411–413, with permission of Macmillan Publishing Company, © 1989.

modify future classes. You also may want to keep records on each individual and assist each one in charting his or her progress.

Another method of simple evaluation is to use pre- and post-program measures, such as brief pencil-and-paper questionnaires to measure knowledge or skill level at the beginning and end of a series of classes. Self-testing and recording may be used. A cost-effective and valid self-administered walking pre-test is the Rockport Walking Test, which establishes a baseline measure for each participant. Some class leaders prefer to use pre-, post-, and follow-up measures. Follow-up can be done by telephone, post card, or home visitation at one month, six months, nine months, and one year after the class—if compliance is being tracked.

Another method is for individual participants to keep weekly charts or logs of their behavior. These should be provided by the leader with stamped, self-addressed envelopes. Reminder telephone calls to mail the weekly log or chart are a must. Buddy systems can also be established, or the leader may want to engage staff in making the telephone calls.

PROGRAM EVALUATION BY THE PARTICIPANTS

If your program is a series with regularly attending participants, time should be given for evaluation during the last session. Evaluation forms should be brief and to the point. Experience has shown that open-ended questions are not as readily answered as are multiple choice questions. For example:

How would you rate this class overall?

1	2	3	4	5
Interesting		OK	Not interesting	

If you ask which topics were most useful, list them with a space for a check mark. Participants may not remember all the topics discussed.

It is important to include evaluative questions that focus on barriers. For example, a large number of negative responses to questions such as, "Did you find it difficult to come to the center?" may help you to acquire funding for transportation or volunteers for other efforts. Do not short-change yourself. Use evaluations to their maximum benefit.

In summary, think evaluation when planning your program. What are your overall goals, and can they be measured? Can you possibly establish a bona fide research project from your preliminary efforts (i.e., use your program as a pilot study)? Can you measure parameters, particularly with regard to exercise, to show improvement? Will this improvement (or maintenance, if that is the goal) fuel compliance efforts by the individual? Evaluation is the cornerstone of building an improved program. Take advantage of it. Learn the skills necessary to do it correctly, and enjoy it. Table 33-1 has been included for your benefit. This checklist is a vital assessment tool necessary prior to the start-up of any program. Using it will enhance overall program success.

BIBLIOGRAPHY

Piscopo, John. *Fitness and Aging.* New York: Macmillan Publishing Company, 1989.

About the Authors

Carole B. Lewis, M.S.G., M.P.A., P.T., Ph.D., has been a physical therapist since 1975. Currently the Chairperson of the Section on Geriatrics of the American Physical Therapy Association, Dr. Lewis has worked in home health care, long-term care, acute care hospitals, rehabilitation departments, and outpatient clinics. Before starting private practice in Washington, D.C., in 1981, she was the director of physical therapy at the Arthritis Rehabilitation Center. In 1979, Dr. Lewis received her two master's degrees in health care management and gerontology from the University of Southern California, and, in 1983, she received her Ph.D. from the University of Maryland.

Dr. Lewis also has extensive publications in the field of gerontology. She has edited a textbook, *Aging: Health Care Challenge, Interdisciplinary Assessment and Treatment of the Geriatric Patient.* In addition, she is currently editing a quarterly journal from Aspen Publishers, Inc. entitled, *Topics in Geriatric Rehabilitation.* Her second textbook, *Improving Mobility for Older Persons,* is available from Aspen Publications.

Finally, Dr. Lewis was honored as one of the ten Outstanding Young Women in America in 1984. She travels extensively as an international lecturer.

Linda C. Campanelli, M.S., Ph.D., has been training exercise leaders and teaching exercise classes since 1976. She began her career in health education and gerontology in Montreal, Canada, her home town, where she taught exercise classes in three languages (English, French, and Italian). Dr. Campanelli continued her studies in gerontology at the University of Maryland, where she received her master's degree in exercise physiology and her doctorate in health education; both graduate degrees were accompanied by a certificate in gerontology.

Dr. Campanelli is presently an assistant professor in the Department of Health and Fitness at The American University, in Washington, D.C. She is also on the faculty of the University of Maryland's University College Institute for Gerontological Practice and The Nursing Home Administrator's 100 Hour Certification Program. She has also been a worksite Health Promotion Site Manager for American Telephone and Telegraph, as well as the former Project Director of the National Center for Health

Promotion and Aging, of the National Council on the Aging.

In addition to her work on the executive committee and board of directors of the Alzheimer's Association of Greater Washington, Dr. Campanelli is presently active in delivering preretirement health education seminars to federal agencies and corporations. She has published articles and chapters in the areas of theories on aging, eldercare, exercise, and death education, as well as lectured internationally.